# Anxiety in a risk society

Few would dispute that we are living at a time of high anxiety and uncertainty in which many of us will experience a crisis of identity at some point or another. At the same time, news media provide us with a daily catalogue of disasters from around the globe to remind us that we inhabit a world of crisis, insecurity and hazard. *Anxiety in a risk society*:

- looks at the problem of contemporary anxiety from a sociological perspective
- highlights its significance for the ways we make sense of risk and uncertainty
- argues that the relationship between anxiety and risk hinges on the nature of anxiety.

Iain Wilkinson believes that there is much for sociologists to learn from those who have made the condition of anxiety the focus of their life's work. By making the problem of anxiety the focus of sociological inquiry, a critical vantage point can be gained from which to attempt an answer to the question: Are we more anxious because we are more 'risk conscious'? This is an original and thought-provoking contribution to the understanding of late modernity as a risk society.

**Iain Wilkinson** is a lecturer in Sociology at the University of Plymouth.

# HEALTH, RISK AND SOCIETY

**Series editor**
Graham Hart
*MRC Social and Public Health Sciences Unit, Glagsow*

In recent years, social scientific interest in risk has increased enormously. In the health field, risk is seen as having the potential to bridge the gap between individuals, communities and the larger social structure, with a theoretical framework which unifies concerns around a number of contemporary health issues. This new series will explore the concept of risk in detail, and address some of the most active areas of current health and research practice.

Previous titles in the series:

# Anxiety in a risk society

Iain Wilkinson

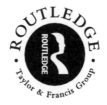

London and New York

First published 2001
by Routledge
11 New Fetter Lane, London EC4P 4EE

Simultaneously published in the USA and Canada
by Routledge
29 West 35th Street, New York, NY 10001

*Routledge is an imprint of the Taylor & Francis Group*

© 2001 Iain Wilkinson

Typeset in Times by M Rules
Printed and bound in Great Britain by
TJ International Ltd, Padstow, Cornwall

*British Library Cataloguing in Publication Data*
A catalogue record for this book is available from the British Library

*Library of Congress Cataloging in Publication Data*
Wilkinson, Iain, 1969–
    Anxiety in a risk society/Iain Wilkinson.
        p. cm. – (Health, risk and society)
    Includes bibliographical references and index.
    I. Risk–Sociological aspects.  2. Anxiety–Sociological aspects.
    I. Title.  II. Series.
    HM1101 W55 2001
    302'.12–dc21                                        00-046013

ISBN 0-415-22680-5 (hbk)
ISBN 0-415-22681-3 (pbk)

# Contents

# Preface

Anxiety, like fear, joy and melancholy, is that most individual of feelings, but yet one that we all share, to a greater or lesser degree, more or less frequently. Sociology has a long history of analysing what appear to be individual ills in terms of the social conditions in which they arise. Durkheim demonstrated how the very personal decision to end one's own life is in fact patterned by culture, and suicide is a social as well as individual phenomenon. In the same vein, Brown and Harris investigated the social aetiology of depression in working-class women, and this too proved to be highly associated with social structural location, and life circumstances and events. Iain Wilkinson continues this tradition with his study of anxiety, both in its aetiology and in responses to it, but goes further than this in his interrogation of the way in which the term has been employed (and sometimes appropriated) by social theorists in recent years, most particularly in the literature on risk. Demonstrating beyond any doubt that anxiety is not the exclusive provenance of psychology or psychiatry, Wilkinson brings to the subject a clarity of thought and writing which renders his arguments a pleasure to read (even though the topic is at the core of our daily concerns and troubles). Seeking to connect what C. Wright Mills identified as the public sphere of structure with the personal realm of experience, he demonstrates that anxiety is both a function of larger changes in society and of the individual experience of un-ease: 'anxiety is conceived not so much as a personality defect, but rather, as a . . . consequence of the social predicaments and cultural contradictions in which individuals . . . live out their day-to-day lives'.

While Wilkinson alerts us to the continuing prescience and insights of the psychoanalytic writings of Freud and Fromm, it is difficult to separate his purpose in this book – of using the social theories of risk to better understand anxiety – from the efforts of others over 150 years to analyse our responses to the entire project of modernity. Durkheim's work on suicide was in the context of a larger issue, the constituents and causes of anomie – literally, normlessness, or an absence of guidance and sense of what is true and right. Marx in his early writing grappled with alienation, and was clear that this was an individual as well as a social condition. Even Weber's preoccupation with *Verstehen* (more properly translated as 'meaning' rather than 'understanding') was an attempt to confront the existential challenge to the individual of a bureaucratised social world. While anomie, alienation and the striving for meaning in social life are not immediately synonymous with anxiety, this engagement with and attempt to understand the distress experienced by people faced with an uncertain present and future are a common feature of an established sociology of industrialisation, and indeed of modernity, a tradition that today we associate with Beck, Giddens and Bauman. But if one were to choose, it is an echo of Weber that resonates most strongly in Wilkinson's book, when he refers to our anxieties as being associated with 'the conviction that there is a deficit of meaning in the world'. By holding out the hope, and alerting us to the value, of the discourses of risk as a means of articulating and addressing the nature of anxiety, Iain Wilkinson does us a major service in clarifying the social meaning, parameters and constituents of this most individual of emotional experiences.

Graham Hart
Series Editor
*Health, Risk and Society*

# Acknowledgements

I am grateful to Ray Pahl for encouraging me to write this book and for all his helpful advice. Special thanks are due to David Morgan for his inspiring conversations and friendship. Many thanks also to my editor, Graham Hart, for his support throughout this project. I dedicate this book to Anna, whose love sustains me.

# Acknowledgements

# Introduction

It is only during the last century that, as a matter of popular understanding, we have begun to explicitly refer to our symptoms of distress in terms of the 'problem of anxiety' (May 1977: 3–19). While history records that people have always worried about the future, and that being emotionally burdened with the stress of life is an elemental feature of the human condition, for us to openly identify some of our more unpleasant feelings as 'anxiety' is almost an exclusively modern phenomenon. Certainly, it is only during the course of the twentieth century that we have begun to specifically diagnose the problems of human psychology as being rooted in our ability to solve the riddles which anxiety poses in our lives. Accordingly, the development of an expansive literature on anxiety reflects a growing preoccupation with understanding the inner self and its ability to cope with the mental and emotional distress of life in modern societies. Moreover, it appears that there are many who hold to the view that such developments imply that the actual *quality* of social life in the twentieth century is considerably worse than that of other periods of human history. While we are living in an age where more people than ever before enjoy good physical health, material prosperity and a great wealth of cultural riches, it is doubtful whether being 'modern' guarantees more happiness. Indeed, many would agree with Emile Durkheim's contention that 'there is no longer any reason for asking whether happiness grows with civilization', rather, it has become all too clear that 'if we are open to more pleasures, we are also open to more pain' (Durkheim 1964: 233–55).

Sociologists have always been keenly aware of the fact that at the same time as modernity may be conceived as 'progress', large numbers of people have been prone to experience their quality of life as something deeply unpleasant. Those associated with the classical legacy of the discipline developed a prodigious range of vocabularies to analyse the components of our unhappiness, and while none of them devoted explicit attention to the problem of anxiety, it is clearly implied within their accounts of the insecurities, stresses and strains of our emergence as 'modern' people. Karl Marx understood capitalist labour relations to intensify a state of alienation which, among other things, was characterised by a state of mind in which workers experience a loss of identity and a sense of homelessness (Marx 1977: 80). Georg Simmel explained the blasé attitude, characteristic of 'metropolitan man', as a psychological defence mechanism against the threat of nervous exhaustion (Simmel 1950: 409–24). Moreover, at a more general level of analysis he understood the cultural dynamics of modernity to involve us in a form of life in which we were more likely to encounter the threat of meaninglessness and agitated states of uncertainty (Simmel 1997: 55–107). A similar 'anxiety of emptiness and meaninglessness' (Tillich 1952: 53–8) is resonant within Max Weber's essays where he addresses the cultural fate of a society 'characterised by rationalization, intellectualization, and above all the disenchantment of the world' (Weber 1948: 155). Indeed, Weber famously conceived such anxiety, as mediated within the culture of Reformation Calvinism, to have provided a vital spur towards the development of 'the spirit of capitalism' (Weber 1958). Perhaps Emile Durkheim comes closest to an explicit sociological conception of anxiety in his account of the anomic personality characterised by a state of emotion which is 'over-excited and freed from all constraint', and which has a sense of being 'lost in the infinity of desires' whereby one is prone to develop a 'passion', [which] no longer recognizing bounds, has no goals left' (Durkheim 1952: 287).

Rollo May records that it is only since the 1930s that the social sciences have begun to devote explicit attention to the problem of anxiety (May 1977: 9–19). This may be explained largely with reference to the influence of Freudian psychoanalysis upon the intellectual culture of Western societies. Sigmund Freud identified anxiety as the 'nodal point at which the most important questions converge [and] a riddle whose solution would be bound to throw a light on our whole mental existence' (Freud 1991: 441). Accordingly, it is in the wake of the revolutionary impact of his thinking that, above all else, psychology has come to be associated with the task of explaining and treating the problems of personality as 'anxiety disorders'. Moreover, where Freud turned to consider the role of culture and society in the development of these problems, sociologists began to take a more explicit interest in the extent to which social processes and cultural developments should be held responsible for making people vulnerable to experience a high state of anxiety as a 'normal' fact of everyday life. In 'Civilization and its Discontents' (1929) he raises the disquieting suggestion that entire epochs of civilisation or possibly even the whole of humanity have become neurotic under the pressure of civilising trends (Freud 1985: 338). Such an opinion has since become commonplace within the literature of sociology. In every decade there have been writers who have openly concurred with the view that there is something deeply wrong with the basic quality of social life in modern societies, and further, that as a matter of explicit concern, increasing numbers of people would identify the problem of anxiety as a major burden of their experience of day-to-day life.

Erich Fromm, Max Horkheimer, Theodor Adorno and Herbert Marcuse all took a working interest in Freud's reading of our discontents within their respective analyses of the alienated condition of humanity when subjected to modern processes of individuation (Jay 1973: 86–112; Bocock 1978: 147–75). In a similar vein, David Riesman in *The Lonely Crowd* (1961) conceived the dominant social character of his times to be defined by an experience of 'diffuse anxiety'. At a more popular level of discussion, C. Wright Mills recognised the brute facts of war, unemployment, family breakdown, chaotic urban life and economic instability as all being among the structural factors giving rise to a social experience of day-to-day life in which the majority of people were troubled with a sense of uneasiness and anxiety, which in its most exteme forms produced 'a deadly unspecified malaise' (Mills 1959: 3–13). Likewise, Peter Berger and colleagues understood modernisation to have exacted a heavy toll upon the collective psyche by creating social conditions in which most people are liable to experience an anguished sense of 'homelessness' (Berger *et al.* 1973). Indeed, following the publication of Auden's *The Age of Anxiety* (1948), which recorded the existential crisis of a generation living in the midst of world war, there has been no shortage of commentators who have recognised the title of this work as a fitting epitaph for the prevailing consciousness of modern times (Tillich 1952: 44; McLuhan 1964: 5; Fromm 1970: 13; Lader 1974; Dunant and Porter 1996; Hollway and Jefferson 1997).

Most would agree that the twentieth century was a time of high anxiety. Moreover, it is commonly accepted that, rather than learning to cope with such conditions, we are in fact becoming more vulnerable to experiencing our world as a place of threatening uncertainty. Within the literature of contemporary sociology the last quarter of a century is now generally represented as a cultural period in which a growing 'sense of crisis' (Noble 1982) has resulted in a

'social state of mind' which is pessimistic to the point of 'paralysing despera-
tion' (Bailey 1988). According to Joe Bailey, 'we have got used to talking as
though the future is not only provisional but is dominated by dangers rather than
opportunities' (ibid.: 1). The culture of 'postmodernism', which has been widely
identified as a collective expression of the intellectual frustration, creative
exhaustion and moral bankruptcy of the modern era, is represented by a number
of commentators as a form of *fin-de-siècle* neurosis (Jay 1988; Kumar 1995;
Meštrović 1991; 1993). For example, Arthur Kroker and David Cook suggest
that 'the postmodern scene' displays an overhwelming sense of panic in face
of the conviction that:

> we are living in a waiting period, a dead space, which [is] marked by
> increasing and random outbursts of political violence, schizoid behav-
> iours, and the implosion of all signs of communication as western
> culture runs down towards the brilliant illumination of a final burnout.
>
> (Kroker and Cook 1988: vii)

Likewise, Zygmunt Bauman understands the postmodern state of mind, among
other things, as a reaction to an experience of society in which the majority of
people live 'under the constant condition of anxiety' whereby they are prone to
become 'neurotic about matters of security' (Bauman 1993: 235).

While the majority of people in contemporary Western societies have had no
direct experience of the ravages of war, in 1996 a collection of essays were published under the same title as Auden's epic poem, which sought to identify the
final decade of the twentieth century as a period in which the modern condition
of anxiety reached a point of feverish intensity. As far as these writers are concerned, the social disruptions connected with the rapid development of
information technology, the burgeoning environmental crisis, unemployment,
job insecurity, the spread of AIDS, the breakdown of moral communities, the
demise of the nuclear family, the crime rate, graphic portrayals of violence in
the media, and even the cultural significance of a new millennium should all be
recognised as factors contributing towards the onset of our current 'exaggerated'
state of anxiety (Dunant and Porter 1996). Over the last decade it has become
a matter of sociological common sense to explicitly identify the society of late
twentieth-century modernity as having a culture of high anxiety which borders
on a state of outright panic (Furedi 1997). Moreover, few would dispute Ray
Pahl's contention that if sociologists are to make any worthwhile contribution to
our understanding of social life in the next century, then this must be made relevant to the fact that the majority of individuals now devote considerable

amounts of time and energy to the effort of coping with the problems which anxiety brings to their lives (Pahl 1995: 1–20).

It is in this context that the topic of risk has risen to prominence in Western social science. Particularly since the publication of Ulrich Beck's seminal 'Risk Society' thesis (1992), increasing numbers of sociologists have come to recognise the high anxieties of late twentieth-century society as being intimately connected with the extent to which we are becoming more 'risk conscious'. Accordingly, it is now understood that we have become culturally disposed to express our anxieties in the language of risk, or conversely, it is through the cultural production of a new knowledge of the risks we face that our lives are conceived as having acquired a new quality of insecurity. Either way, it is commonly assumed that the more we recognise ourselves as being 'at risk', the more vulnerable we become towards anxiety.

It is by theorising the interrelationship between social perceptions of risk and the experience of anxiety that sociologists are now seeking to endow their work with the power to reveal the connections between the cultural logic of Western modernity and the feeling that something is deeply wrong with the quality of our experience of day-to-day life. Deborah Lupton introduces a recent review of the sociological literature on risk, with the suggestion that this word is now understood by many 'to stand as one of the focal points of feelings of fear, anxiety and uncertainty' (Lupton 1999a: 12). Among other things, the sociology of risk is involved in both promoting and critically evaluating a cultural narrative on modernity which identifies the current *fin-de-siècle* as a period obsessively preoccupied with the conviction that we are living under the threat of hazardous uncertainty. Accordingly, by attempting to discern the origins of 'risk consciousness' and by venturing to explain the social distribution of perceptions of risk, sociologists now offer a means of accounting for the cultural dynamics of anxiety and its origins within the social constitution of late modernity.

This wholly negative association between social perceptions of risk and the experience of anxiety is perhaps surprising in light of the fact that for most of its history, one was more likely to come across 'risk' as a principle of insurance, a gambling stake or a business opportunity. In this context, 'risk' is an abstract term invoking a probabilistic calculus for establishing the most cost-effective and financially lucrative means of dealing with a hazardous world. To negotiate the future in terms of risk implied a willingness to place our trust in the powers of reason and a confidence in our technological mastery of nature (de Roover 1945; Jackson 1989). Accordingly, the economic historian, Peter Bernstein, recognises the possibility of 'taking risks' as one of the principal technological and intellectual achievements of the modern age (Bernstein 1998). By contrast, sociologists maintain that in the present cultural climate, the concept of 'risk' is losing its positive connections with wealth and opportunity and, rather, is being used exclusively to evoke the threat hazard, the fear of damage, the failure of 'progress' and a loss of confidence in the security of the world. As far as the majority of sociological commentators are concerned, the current prominence of the language of 'risk' cannot be explained in terms of the acquisitive allure of probabilistic thinking, rather, it is generally understood to be related to the fact that people are increasingly disposed to see the world as full of danger (Douglas 1985; 1992; Beck 1992; 1995; 1999; Ewald 1993).

Most obviously the language of risk appears in a daily supply of 'news' which is devoted to cataloguing the fact that we live in a dangerous world. Content analyses of Western newspapers document the fact that throughout the 1990s the word 'risk' was used with increasing frequency as a synonym for 'hazards', 'threats' and 'disasters' (Lupton 1999a: 9–10). The concept of being 'at risk' constantly appears in reports on threats to our health, the hazards of technology, our distrust of governments and our fears of society. Accordingly, sociologists have come to identify our 'mediated' knowledge of 'high-conse-quence risks' as a major source of contemporary anxiety (Giddens 1991), or at least as an expression of a new feeling of insecurity and a state of moral confu-sion that characterises the day-to-day experience of social life in industrial societies (Furedi 1997).

Moreover, the prominence of the language of 'risk' in the public sphere is also connected to the fact that issues of health and safety have become increas-ingly important as part of the activities and organisation of businesses and public utilities (Adams 1995: 31–2). In the past twenty years the assessment and management of risk for the purposes of maximising our protection and security have grown into a multibillion-dollar industry (Freudenberg and Pastor 1992). This may be conceived, in part, as the logical conclusion of a cultural predis-position to make health matters and safe conduct subject to the authority of calculable rules (Luhmann 1993: 28; Skolbekken 1995). However, the majority of commentators place an emphasis upon the extent to which the pursuit of risk reduction relates to the emergence of a society which is obsessively preoccupied with a search for safety. Indeed, the growth of the field of risk research within the social sciences is in large part connected with the extent to which govern-ments and industry, in an effort to avoid costly legal and civil disputes, have become increasingly concerned to understand people's apparently 'irrational' anxieties about new technological developments and their distrust of those in positions of authority. Accordingly, huge investments have been made in the study of risk perception and communication, largely with the aim of 'managing'

conflicting opinions as to the magnitude of hazards and quelling society's para-
noia about issues of public health and personal security.

At present there is no agreement among sociologists as to why we have
latently become so preoccupied with threats to our health and safety, or what
significance we should attach to the popular codification of 'danger' as 'risk'.
Moreover, while it is becoming increasingly clear that people are not all concerned with the same types of risk, considerable controversy surrounds the
possibility of establishing a precise account of the social distribution of risk perception, let alone explaining such a phenomenon (Cutter 1993: 11–32; Boholm
1996; Sjoberg 1997; 1998; 2000; Brenot *et al.* 1998). Indeed, the ways in which
sociologists themselves assess the magnitude of the risks we face appears to
have a decisive bearing upon the ways in which they theorise the social development of 'risk consciousness' and its political significance for the likely futures
which await us (Lupton 1999a: 17–83; Clark and Short 1993). Accordingly, the
majority of commentators structure their work around a defence of their
favoured rendition of the 'reality' of risk, and thereby make considerable efforts
to unmask the ideological biases of opposing points of view. The sociological
industry which has built up around the topic of risk is for the most part concerned to explain the cultural production of our beliefs about health and
technological hazards and their role within the development of a new style of
politics and ethics for a society, which by the 'accidental' side-effects of its own
design, has (depending upon whose 'expert' opinion you trust) increased the
threat of large-scale environmental catastrophe (Lash *et al.* 1996; O'Mahoney
1999).

In this context most sociologists have recognised no need for any detailed
study of anxiety itself. The majority of writers make passing reference to the
fact that 'risk consciousness' is either a cause or expression of anxiety as if this
is to state the obvious. Moreover, having noted this 'fact', their task is conceived
largely in terms of the need to explain the social production and distribution of
contrasting perceptions of risk. Accordingly, the problem of anxiety itself is
generally not recognised as presenting us with any significant conceptual diffi-
culties, and in its own terms is not considered to be in need of any substantive
sociological analysis. However, this book is written under the conviction that
where the meaning of the relationship between 'risk consciousness' and anxiety
is open to a range of conflicting interpretations, then this may be explained in
large part as a consequence of the complexity of the problems which anxiety
brings to our lives. I contend that it is by making the problem of anxiety the
focus of sociological inquiry that a critical vantage point may be established
for making a fuller assessment of the origins and dimensions of 'risk

consciousness'. Furthermore, if the 'sociological imagination' is to use the study of risk as means of helping people 'to understand the larger historical scene in terms of its meaning for the inner life', I maintain that this requires a more detailed demonstration of the precise links between 'the public issues of structure' and the ways in which individuals encounter and cope with anxiety in the contexts of their daily struggles amidst 'the personal troubles of milieu' (Mills 1959: 5–11).

## Aims of the book

This book aims to present the reader with a means of critically assessing the contention that society is more anxious because is it more risk conscious. In order to fulfil this ambition it is written under the direction of two basic objectives: first, by focusing upon the task of conceptualising the specific components of the problem of anxiety, a set of analytical tools are developed for investigating the allegation that society is becoming more anxious. Second, this investigation is brought to a critical focus upon the contention that 'risk consciousness' is the definitive expression and/or cause of an 'exaggerated' condition of anxiety in contemporary societies. I argue that both at the level of conceptual analysis and in the practice of empirical research, the symbolic association between 'risk' and 'anxiety' is open to a range of conflicting interpretations. While 'risk consciousness' can be represented as a cause of anxiety, depending upon the peculiar characteristics of different types of risk, it may more appropriately be conceived as a means whereby people may achieve a symbolic resolution to their problems, or even an opportunity for discharging some of their symptoms of distress. Moreover, where the language of risk appears in our news media, this may be conceived not so much as a reflection of the anxious concerns of 'the public' in general, but rather, as an attempt to co-opt the negative social meaning of anxiety on behalf of the political ambitions of minority concerns.

I attempt a sociological conception of the problem of anxiety which gives due consideration to the analytical complexity of this condition as revealed in the works of those who specialise in the study of personal distress. The particular ontology and phenomenology of anxiety are seldom recognised as being of sociological concern, rather, these are generally understood to comprise the disciplinary interests of psychology and psychiatry. While sociologists have come to debate the social determinants of our modern cultural malaise with explicit reference to the problem of anxiety, to date, there have been few attempts to analyse the condition of anxiety itself so as to attempt a proper demonstration of the presumed relationship between its structural causes and personal affects. While I celebrate the capacity of the sociological imagination to provide us with a means of reflecting critically upon the social structures which govern our lives, the study of anxiety leads me to question its success at conceptualising the interrelationship between public issues and the problems of private life.

There is much for sociologists to learn from those who have made the condition of anxiety the explicit focus of their life's work. Freud warned us that 'anxiety is not . . . a simple matter' (1979: 288) and at the beginning of a new century there is still no consensus when it comes to conceptualising its constituent aspects and there are a range of contrasting and conflicting interpretations of its significance for the human condition. Following Freud's advice, I believe that it is only by being prepared to enter into dialogue with the many theorists and researchers who have analysed the complexity of this phenomenon at the level of individual experience that sociologists might contribute something worthwhile to the ongoing task of finding 'something that will tell us what anxiety really is . . . [or at least] some criterion that will enable us to distinguish true statements about it from false ones' (ibid.). Accordingly in the first part of the book, I focus specifically upon the task of analysing the constituent aspects of anxiety, its social distribution, and the ways in which people cope with the problems it brings to their lives.

In Chapter 1 I discuss the tradition of conceptualising the distinctive attributes of anxiety in contradistinction to fear so as to explain my theoretical commitment towards a definition of anxiety which identifies the problem of definition, and more specifically the problem of self-definition, as the key to understanding the ways in which individuals encounter and struggle to make sense of this experience. In so doing, I present the reader with a conception of anxiety as a reaction to social processes and cultural experiences in which our doubts and uncertainties are encountered as a threat to our personal security and even our identity as a personality. Moreover, while focusing my analysis upon the problem of interpreting the phenomenological or existential meaning of anxiety, I also highlight some of the ways in which sociologists may attempt to explain the anxious condition of modern individuals as a product of the social conflicts and cultural contradictions which comprise their experience of day-to-day life.

In Chapter 2 I provide a critical investigation of the problem of establishing the overall distribution of anxiety in society. Here I am particularly concerned to ask whether it is possible for us to identify who has the most anxiety as well as the social factors which are responsible for making them feel this way. I reflect upon the findings of empirical studies conducted under the auspices of stress research in order to highlight some of the social processes and life events which are understood to be implicated within the development of symptoms of anxiety linked to an episode of mental or physical illness. I argue that where stress research reveals the socially structured contexts in which people are most likely to encounter aetiologically significant experiences of psychological distress, then this may also be considered to provide us with some of the most sociologically 'objective' indicators of anxiety in contemporary societies. However, given the moderating force of symbolic forms of culture upon the negative meanings given to the processes and events which cause us to feel this way, I am also concerned to emphasise the provisional character of all accounts of the prevalence of anxiety at any particular time and place. I understand the social distribution of anxiety to be determined by cultural processes in which there is always scope for individuals to reappraise the meanings of the stressful situations in which they find themselves.

However, where I turn to focus upon the task of coping, in Chapter 3 I am particularly concerned to dwell upon the extent to which our individual inclinations and abilities to endow our lives with positive meaning are liable to be constrained by the social and cultural conditions in which we are made to live. Where in the context of stress research and health psychology, coping thoughts and behaviours are most likely to be represented as matters of individual personality, I emphasise the extent to which these may be identified as an expression of the forms of society, economy and culture in which we find ourselves. Indeed, in order to develop some of the points raised in Chapter 2, I note that those who occupy a social position which restricts access to the prime resources for coping, also tend to display the most severe symptoms of anxiety. Accordingly, I consider the extent to which solutions to the problem of anxiety lie more in the direction of a change to society than in helping individuals to better adapt themselves to the prevailing status quo. In this context, I raise some critical questions with regard to the role of sociology within the political struggle to realise a form of social organisation which is conducive to our mental health and emotional well-being.

In the second part of the book I focus my discussion more directly upon the relationship between 'risk consciousness' and anxiety. Here I aim to highlight the conflicting range of interpretations that might be given to the risk–anxiety relationship. Moreover, I am concerned to offer an explanation for this state of affairs not only with reference to the permutations of risk discourse and debate, but also with an emphasis upon the extent to which all attempts at explaining the problem of anxiety in contemporary societies are liable to be drawn into the realms of speculation. I understand opposing interpretations of the bearing of 'risk consciousness' upon the experience of anxiety not only as a consequence of the range of contrasting meanings which may now be given to the concept of risk, but also as a product of the extent to which the 'objective' dimensions of the condition of anxiety (as opposed to the state of fear), remain shrouded in obscurity. Indeed, the narrative I offer is largely inspired by the contention that where there is always uncertainty in the lived experience of anxiety, then we may be certain that, as a topic of cultural analysis, the 'reality' of this condition will remain open to debate.

In Chapter 4 I examine some of the ways in which the hermeneutics of risk may be used to assess the cultural significance of 'risk consciousness' for the experience of anxiety. I present an overview of the semantics of risk which focuses upon the extent to which the increasing tension between the assurances and uncertainties of risk analysis gives rise to a cultural situation where the precise meaning of this concept is now more open to (political) debate than at any other time in its history. Moreover, where now a conflict of interpretations surrounds the meaning of risk, I aim to explore this in terms of its bearing upon the condition of anxiety in contemporary societies. In this context, I note that where knowledge about risks may sometimes be identified as a cause of anxiety, on other occasions it may serve as a cultural resource for better coping with this condition. Contrasting sociological conceptions of the risk–anxiety relationship tend to place an emphasis on one side or the other of this dichotomy. This is subsequently analysed in relation to political disputes over the reality of 'risk' and opposing sociological perspectives on the rationality of anxiety.

In Chapter 5 I focus my inquiry upon Ulrich Beck's contention that 'the risk society marks the dawning of a speculative age in everyday perception and thought' (Beck 1992: 73). Where the evidence for this is made manifest within academic disputes over the 'reality' of the risk, here I shall ultimately be concerned to dwell upon the extent to which the problem of anxiety itself guarantees that there will be no final certainty, but always speculation, when it comes to accounting for the ways in which people acquire and create meanings for their world in terms of risk. However, in addition to this, and as a means of elaborating upon the theme of speculation, I explore some of the analytical issues which arise in connection with the task of accounting for the cultural dynamics of the interrelationship between media, risk and anxiety. While dwelling upon the inadequacy of our methodological and theoretical frameworks for handling the complexity of processes of symbolic production and exchange, I aim to highlight the extent to which, in the final analysis, the condition of anxiety is liable to ensure that the cultural significance of 'risk consciousness' remains subject to a conflict of interpretations.

Finally, I would add that in writing this book, I have brought together a wide range of literatures, which in many instances were not written with a sociological audience in mind. Accordingly, I apologise in advance to those who consider my selective reinterpretations of different strands of thought confuse (or abuse) the original meanings which authors intended for their works. In what follows, I consider much of my task to involve a work of hermeneutical recovery, but in reviewing some key ideas from our past for structuring the lines of future inquiry, it is perhaps inevitable that while being 're-embedded' in the domain of contemporary sociological discourse their cultural significance is transformed (Thompson 1996).

By returning to explore some of the earliest formulations of the problem of anxiety, I am particularly concerned to trace the historical development of a 'basic vision' (Fromm 1944: 380) of this condition as more a matter of social than personal pathology. While raising a number of 'side issues' for debate, it is largely on the basis of a 'constructive reinterpretation' (ibid.) of anxiety as a sign that something is seriously wrong with the condition of our social world that I aim to present the reader with a form of cultural narrative for understanding the ways in which people may personally experience the 'reality' of a risk society. In so doing, I hope that I may be judged to make progress in clearing a conceptual space for areas of research and debate which to date remain largely neglected within the emergent sociology of risk.

Part I

---

# The problem of anxiety

# Towards a sociological conception of the problem of anxiety

Anxiety is a complex phenomenon, which both at the level of individual experience and as the subject of academic study, concerns points of uncertainty which inevitably give rise to conflicting interpretations and evaluations of its principal causes, defining characteristics and significance for our lives. While our conceptions of this unpleasant part of being human have become more complexly detailed and subtly nuanced, there is still no consensus among researchers as to how far we should recognise anxiety as a normal or inevitable aspect of life in modern societies. Moreover, where we have achieved a greater understanding of the possible causes of this experience, anxiety seems to retain a sense or appearance of indeterminacy which guarantees that its *precise* origins will always remain open to debate. Accordingly, from the outset of our discussion the reader should remain alert to the fact that it is only possible to write on this subject by adopting a selective point of view.

Most researchers in the field of clinical and health psychology now understand the condition of anxiety to be comprised of a complex emotional process which involves not only our thoughts, but also our physiology and behaviour. In this context anxiety is held to consist in the interrelationship between affective experiences, bodily reactions and behavioural responses. For the most part, clinicians have focused upon the task of developing therapies for treating specific types of anxiety disorder which are explained with reference to the personal histories, emotional characteristics, psychologies and physiologies of their patients. A vast amount of research has been conducted into the problem of anxiety conceived as a form of 'neurosis', 'abnormality' or 'pathology', which is caused by the extent to which individuals have been made temperamentally vulnerable to develop modes of cognition and adaptive behavioural/physiological responses which are not normally associated with those of healthy members of society (Edelmann 1992; Rachman 1998).

As far as clinical practice is concerned, the social and cultural components of anxiety have been treated as a marginal concern (Smail 1999). Where behaviourists would refer us to the conditioning influence of a social environment, they have remained largely unmotivated to explain anxiety with any reference to the structural dynamics of modern societies, rather, they have focused upon the task of analysing the psychological and biological mechanisms through which individuals learn maladaptive responses to the 'stimuli' of their immediate surroundings (Eysenck 1957; 1967; Gray 1987). Similarly, where cognitive approaches may lead us to consider the social reproduction and cultural conditioning of the thoughts which preoccupy their patients, researchers have been predominantly concerned to explain how neurotic individuals are made vulnerable to anxiety as a consequence of their own (mis)interpretations and (mis)appraisals of the situations in which they find themselves (Beck *et al.* 1985; Brewin 1996). Moreover, while some of the most celebrated figures within the traditions of psychoanalysis have sought to alert their profession to the influence of social forces and cultural factors upon the development of neurotic personalities, for the most part therapists have conceived their task in terms of helping individuals to come to a new way of 'seeing' their experience of the world so that their problems do not appear to be so great as to prevent them from living a more 'normal' life. Accordingly, rather than looking at the social antagonisms and cultural conflicts which comprise their experience of life in modern societies, clinical psychologists and psychotherapists have been inclined to explain anxiety with an emphasis upon the problems and weaknesses of individuals with neurotic disorders (Smail 1984). On this view, our vulnerability to anxiety is more likely to be understood as a consequence of the developmental trends of our individual personalities rather than those of the cultural conditions and social structures in which we find ourselves.

While I shall make some passing references to this literature, these are selected with the aim of conceiving anxiety not so much as a particular problem for unusual individuals who are perceived as having something 'wrong' with them but, rather, for the purpose of developing a more general conception of anxiety as an occasional experience which is common to us all. Moreover, I shall be particularly concerned to emphasise the extent to which the experience of anxiety may be understood as a product of social processes and cultural values. In this context, it is possible to recognise certain individuals and social groups as being made more vulnerable to anxiety as a consequence of their location within the structure of society and the quality of their commitments towards the dominant cultural values of our times; more precisely, one may begin to develop a conception of the social distribution of different occasions for anxiety, as well as the contrasting ways in which people set about coping with the problems it brings to their lives. Accordingly, I am interested to note the extent to which 'neurotic' symptoms or excessive states of anxiety may be explained in terms of a process of social and cultural determination. From this perspective, anxiety is conceived not so much as a personality defect but, rather, as a function or consequence of the social predicaments and cultural contradictions in which individuals are made to live out their everyday lives.

It is in accordance with this emphasis upon the social reproduction and cultural conditioning of our experience of the world that I shall explain my interest in a definition of anxiety which stresses the extent to which this is inextricably bound to the problem of establishing a proper meaning for situations of foreboding obscurity. Accordingly, I maintain that the experience of anxiety should not only be recognised as being conditioned by the culture of our times but also as a problem of culture. Following commentators such as Erich Fromm (1942; 1947; 1995) and Karen Horney (1937; 1939; 1946; 1950), I conceive the condition of anxiety to be intimately connected with the extent to which the cultural experience of modern societies may sometimes make us feel deeply insecure about our identity and purpose in a world which appears to be deprived of its proper significance and value. The term 'anxiety' is a symbolic form of culture representing a state of mind and emotion by which we are made to be convinced that we are in a situation of threatening uncertainty. However, we should also recognise that being made to think and feel this way takes place in relation to the extent to which we lack, or rather, are denied the cultural resources for conceiving a means of escaping the suspected course of our fate.

For the purpose of maintaining a clear analytical distinction between anxiety and other distressing states of emotion such as fear, shame, and humiliation, I hold to the view that we are only kept in anxiety for so long as we remain overwhelmed by the sense that we lack a sufficient means of knowing how to keep ourselves from harm's way. Moreover, I understand anxiety to function to alert us to the fact that it is precisely due to our ignorance that we are at risk of being damaged, hurt, and humiliated. Accordingly, insofar as it keeps us traumatised under the conviction that we have yet to find a proper meaning for the threatening situations in which we find ourselves, anxiety forces us to keep searching for a means of knowing how to think and what to do in face of an unknown quantity of danger. With this in mind, I would argue that insofar as we are committed to defining the meaning of the phenomenological experience of anxiety, then we are liable to come across the paradox that it seems to be borne by consciousness as a problem of definition; so long as anxiety remains, we are left frustrated in the knowledge that our culture has yet to provide us with a capacity to understand the 'true' significance of our feelings of distress, and further, it has yet to equip us with a sufficient means of overcoming, or avoiding, the sense of being overwhelmed by the threatening uncertainty of the possible futures which await us.

This chapter begins with a more detailed attempt to define the problem of anxiety in terms of the distressing obscurity which dominates the subjective experience of being held captive by this condition. I then go on to discuss the social meaning of anxiety in the context of a theoretical analysis of the distinction between anxiety and fear. Accordingly, I explain my bias towards a definition of anxiety which conceives this to be part of the experience in which individuals struggle to come to terms with the threatening sense of meaninglessness and states of helplessness which comprise their symptoms of social distress. I highlight some of the ways in which psychologists have conceived the social and cultural components of this experience as a means of introducing the basic tenets of a sociological conception of anxiety. At this point, I offer a brief account of some of the major theoretical themes which characterise the sociological discourse on anxiety. In this context, I attempt to explain how a process of 'individualisation', the loss of community and tradition, and the modern experience of work and employment are all conceived as having contributed towards the development of a social environment in which we are made vulnerable to the distress of anxiety.

## The problem of definition

While few would doubt the importance of anxiety as a defining characteristic of our humanity, there is certainly no agreement as to how one should interpret its significance for the development and well-being of our psychology, interpersonal relations and culture. Indeed, researchers cannot even agree upon how to describe the main components of the experience of anxiety, let alone reach a consensus as to the factors which make us more or less vulnerable to being in this condition. Any attempt to define or explain 'the problem of anxiety' is liable to court controversy. However, perhaps this is precisely what we should expect for it appears that the *experience* of anxiety always leaves us struggling to make sense of its true origins and purposes.

There is a persistent conflict of interpretations as to the proper definition of anxiety. Indeed, William Fischer advises that we should expect to find that 'there are as many conceptions of anxiety as there are theories of man' (Fischer 1970: 135). This may be understood not only as the result of the outwardly observable complexity of the phenomena of this condition, but also as a consequence of the fact that the sensible quality of the inner experience of anxiety is borne by consciousness as a problem of meaning which invites, or rather, demands us to engage in a speculative search for its 'true' origins and identity. Accordingly, I am inclined to believe that the distressing obscurity which comprises the experience of being the victim of anxiety may be held partly responsible for the ongoing academic debate over its constituent aspects and precise causes.

When held captive by the experience of being in anxiety, individuals commonly express an elevated sense of threatening uncertainty. They appear to have difficulty in establishing a sufficiently clear conception of the causes of their complaint, or the proper identity of an anticipated danger, and thereby are given over to an unpleasant feeling of uneasy suspense. Among other things, when caught by the state of anxiety, individuals are made to be distressed by the extent to which they conceive themselves to be in a dangerous situation yet do not know how to think and what to do in order to protect themselves. Indeed, it appears that it is by so traumatising us with the knowledge of our own ignorance that anxiety functions to alert us to, and prepare us for, the threat of danger (Freud 1979: 324–9). So long as we are in anxiety, we are troubled by the conviction that something important remains to be known so that we can avoid being in harm's way, and thereby, so long as we do not fall into despair, we are driven to search for ideal and practical solutions to the problems it impresses upon our consciousness.

Accordingly, it appears that where there is anxiety there is always a problem of definition; anxiety always presents us and leaves us with agonising questions as to its precise significance and purpose. We are kept in anxiety so long as we are left struggling to define the threatening situation in which we find ourselves. Anxiety is aroused in social contexts where individuals suspect themselves to be in a threatening situation, but nevertheless, are still deprived of the knowledge which is sufficient to reveal enough about the causes of their complaint so that they can take the necessary steps to avoid the danger. On this basis, following the pioneering accounts of Søren Kierkegaard (1980) and

Sigmund Freud (1979), theorists have traditionally held to the view that the problem of definition should occupy the centre of any attempt to define and explain the meaning of anxiety. Moreover, it is also understood that as we acquire a greater knowledge of the proper dimensions of an anticipated danger, then we should also be relieved from the tension of anxiety. However, it is important to add that where knowledge frees us from anxiety, it may only bring us so far as to realise the proper identity of our fears.

As a matter of conceptual analysis, it is suggested that where fears 'refer to something definite' (Kierkegaard 1980: 42), by contrast anxiety, has 'a quality of indefiniteness and lack of object' (Freud 1979: 325). Fears have a specific focus whereby individuals are held to have a clear understanding of the object which they endeavour to avoid, however, the object of anxiety may be recognised as the paradox that it is 'the negation of every object' (Tillich 1952: 45). Where fear always has something in its sights, the distinctiveness of anxiety lies in the fact that, precisely speaking, it appears to be directed towards nothing (Kierkegaard 1980: 43). Consequently, when caught by anxiety, we are distressed by our inability to recognise the causes of our condition for they remain hidden in obscurity. Moreover, anxiety leaves us powerless to deliver ourselves from our fate, since there is nothing upon which we can concentrate our energies.

Nevertheless, insofar as they may be identified as consisting of a relationship of mutual dependency, it is not always easy to maintain a clear distinction between fear and anxiety. Where we are afraid of a definite something such as pain, being a failure, a lack of recognition or losing something of great value or somebody loved, our anxieties arise in connection with the threatening uncertainty of not knowing how we should be, or what we should do in anticipation of these awful events. Anxiety feeds upon the unknown elements of our fears. Moreover, aside from the harms which they bring, what makes our fears so terrible may be due to the fact that they are the route towards anxiety. Indeed, Paul Tillich suggests that the 'sting of fear is anxiety' insofar as we may be most tormented by the terrible anticipation of its possible implications for our lives (Tillich 1952: 46).

Accordingly, the key to explaining the difference between fear and anxiety is represented as amounting to a difference in the amount or quality of knowledge we possess as to the objective dimensions of an anticipated danger. At the same time as anxiety anticipates an experience of helplessness, it leaves us helplessly searching to find an object which is sufficient to translate our anxieties into fear (Freud 1979: 326–7). It appears that anxiety thrives upon the tension between our knowledge and ignorance of fearful situations. Moreover, it is understood that as we acquire a fuller understanding of the actual causes of our condition we shall reach a position in which the vague uncertainties of anxiety are transformed into the known objects of fear. Thus, Paul Tillich contends that so long as we are in a state of anxiety our minds become a 'factory of fear', because it is only when we have successfully translated our anxieties into fears that we may take the necessary steps to avoid and protect ourselves from an anticipated danger (Tillich: 1952: 47). Similarly, Rollo May emphasises that for those beset by the problem of anxiety, it is the sense of agonising uncertainty which is so traumatically threatening since, 'one cannot fight what one does not know' (May 1977: 207). Accordingly, Stanley Rachman notes that psychotherapists have traditionally held to the assumption that it is by converting anxiety into fear that they may help their patients to better manage their symptoms of emotional distress. For example, Freud maintained that it was by acquiring a knowledge of the object of an anticipated danger that he sought to enable his patients to remove themselves from the trauma of neurotic anxiety (Freud 1979: 324–9). Such a motive implies that 'anxiety is not-fear [sic] simply by reason of default; that is, we have anxiety when the focus of fear is elusive' (Rachman 1998: 7). By liberating patients from the uncertainty of the causes of their affliction, it is considered a 'progressive step' to have helped them to move from the condition of anxiety into the state of fear.

However, at this point in my discussion, the reader should be aware of the fact that I have become embroiled in theoretical commitments which are far removed from any simple or uncontested definition of the problem of anxiety. Indeed, where researchers analyse the problem of anxiety in terms of the activity of our nervous system, a type of expressive behaviour, or the cognitive structuring of our emotions, then the distinction between anxiety and fear tends to be treated as largely irrelevant to the task of explaining how our bodies, minds and behaviour combine to provide us with different kinds of emotional experience (Edelmann 1992: 1–18). Moreover, in the field of experimental psychology there are writers who use these terms interchangeably when analysing the neurophysiological and behavioural components of different types of phobia and anxiety disorder (Mowrer 1939; Fischer 1970: 50–9). Accordingly, I would draw attention to the fact that the tradition of defining anxiety in contradistinction to fear appears most prominently within the works of those concerned to advance a means of interpreting the phenomenological or existential meaning of the overall quality of this experience. It is especially in this context that we are also more likely to find psychologists taking an interest in the cultural components of anxiety and its wider significance for our social experience of day-to-day life.

## The social meaning of anxiety

Where psychologists take an interest in the social meaning of anxiety they are usually most committed to upholding the analytical distinction between anxiety and fear. For example, Harry Stack Sullivan recognises anxiety to have a social meaning which is quite different to that of fear. He argues that fear is an adaptive response to dangerous situations which we hold in common with other animals. Fear functions to mobilise our bodies for action whereby we might flee the environmental situation or object which threatens to do harm to our physical existence (Sullivan 1953: 50). Moreover, fears are understood to hold no necessary significance for our sociability. By contrast, Sullivan places a special emphasis upon 'the interpersonal nature of anxiety' (Sullivan 1964: 297). He conceives anxiety to be exclusively linked to the social achievement of presenting and knowing oneself as an adequate human being. He maintains that anxiety is aroused exclusively in relation to the experience of social disapproval, and in its most extreme forms, it serves to make us acutely aware of our anticipated 'embarrassment, shame, humiliation, guilt and chagrin' before others (ibid.: 318). The distinctive sign of being in anxiety is that individuals are not so much motivated by the drive to escape their environment or any particular object, rather, they have a desperate need to flee from themselves. Thus in this definition, anxiety, unlike fear, has no object insofar as it is understood to be rooted in the unbearable experience of being the subject of social failure (Fischer 1970: 33–4).

Similarly, Rollo May argues that the term 'anxiety' should be especially reserved to describe those experiences which threaten the possibility of maintaining oneself as a personality. Accordingly, where the specific focus of fear may cause us harm, it is nevertheless considered to lack the capacity to destroy the basic values which comprise the meaning of our humanity. By contrast, he emphasises that 'what will always be true in anxiety is that the threat is to a value held by that particular individual to be essential to his existence and, consequently, to his security as a personality' (May 1977: 206). To illustrate his point, May refers to a case study of a patient, 'Tom', who considered committing suicide when threatened with unemployment. The meaning of Tom's life was heavily dependent upon his capacity to fulfil his role as a breadwinner; to be denied this role was tantamount to losing his sense of purpose and identity (ibid.). Accordingly, for May, a particular emphasis should be placed upon the negative cultural value of the threatening uncertainty of the situation which arouses the experience of anxiety. Moreover, in common with Sullivan, but with a different emphasis, May considers the fact that anxiety attacks the very foundations of our personality to provide the explanation for why it is encountered as an 'objectless experience'. He writes:

> [T]he objectless nature of anxiety arises from the fact that the security base of the individual is threatened, and since it is in terms of this security base that the individual has been able to experience himself as a self in relation to objects, the distinction between subject and object also breaks down.
>
> (May 1977: 208)

A particular focus upon the subjective meaning of anxiety in the context of our social experience of the cultural conflicts and contradictions of modern societies is also to be found in the works of Karen Horney (1937; 1939; 1946; 1950). Moreover, she is similarly inclined to emphasise the extent to which anxiety takes place where we are made vulnerable to experiences of social hostility which undermine our sense of purpose and our feeling of identity. Where we clearly know what to do about our fears, Horney conceives the experience of anxiety to be particularly associated with a sense of meaninglessness and helplessness which threatens to destroy the very core of our personalities (1939: 193–5). She describes the 'basic anxiety' which characterises the cultural experience of modernity as 'a feeling of being small, insignificant, helpless, deserted, endangered, in a world that is out to abuse, cheat, attack, humiliate, betray [and] envy' (1937: 92). Again, an emphasis is being placed on the extent to which anxiety is encountered within the unbearable experience of being the subject of failure, hostility and conflict. Furthermore, it is also held to involve a profound sense of disorientation as well as a struggle for safety, meaning and self-identity.

In the works of these three theorists, a special emphasis is placed not so much upon the physical experience and behavioural components of anxiety, but rather, upon the subjective experience of the threat of meaninglessness and helplessness. Accordingly, a clear distinction between fear and anxiety is maintained on the grounds that, strictly speaking, it is only the latter which is specifically related to the fact that our humanity is comprised by the social task of establishing and sustaining a *meaningful* relationship towards others, ourselves and our physical environment. Moreover, where psychologists have highlighted the importance of conceptualising the subjective experience of anxiety as being intimately related to the problem of meaning, they have tended to become more interested in matters of sociology as a means of detecting the origins of this experience.

For example, both Horney and May make explicit attempts to develop their work in this direction. Rollo May maintains that 'there is reason for assuming that individual competitive success is both the dominant goal in our culture and the most pervasive occasion for anxiety' (May 1977: 177). He suggests that a society which places a pressure upon individuals to succeed in a competitive market for wealth and prestige is liable to give rise to social institutions in which individuals encounter one another in relationships of mutual hostility. Accordingly, their anxiety tends to be closely associated with a social experience of isolation and an aggressive striving for success. Moreover, for the majority of people, the most obvious solution to the sense of worthlessness and powerlessness that comprises the experience of anxiety is to maximise their efforts to attain a position of competitive advantage, for they have been conditioned into the belief that it is by achieving the social recognition of being a successful person that they shall acquire a sense of personal dignity and the power to direct the course of their lives. Thus, he conceives the most commonly accepted solution to anxiety as also the major cause of this problem; the struggle to achieve success gives rise to a 'vicious circle' of ever increasing anxiety (ibid.: 231–9).

Karen Horney also draws attention to the fact that the economies of modern societies are based upon an ideological principle of competitive individualism which is liable to exacerbate the hostilities between human beings. Accordingly, she understands all of us to participate in a cultural experience where we are made vulnerable to feel a deep sense of insecurity as well as the awful tension that derives from the fear of failure. Moreover, she suggests that we are likely to find ourselves emotionally frustrated as a consequence of our social relationships being impaired by a constant struggle to gain superiority, prestige and economic security. Horney highlights a number of cultural contradictions which, according to their frequency and intensity, she conceives as being a major cause of the anxiety which disposes individuals to adopt 'neurotic' attitudes and behaviours. Aside from the basic contradiction between the competitive search for success and an ethic of brotherly love and humility, she notes that since there appears to be no end to the material ambitions of modern individuals they will always be liable to come across a discrepancy between their consumer desires and the possibility of having these needs fulfilled. Furthermore, the popular belief in the freedom of the individual to achieve whatever they desire on the basis of their own energies and hard work, tends to be contradicted by the constraints of social position, the competitive force of others and by the fact that we live in a world of limited resources and restricted opportunities. All these contradictions are held to be a major source of anxiety and, where they are most accentuated, she claims that individuals are liable to develop 'neurotic character traits' in response to the tensions which this condition imposes upon their lives (Horney 1937: 281–90).

By taking up such issues, Horney and May identify an important role for sociology within the study of anxiety and neuroses. Horney urges psychoanalysts to bring their work under the influence of sociology so as to link the structure of neuroses to the social structuring of cultural processes. Moreover, she commends sociology as a means of understanding why certain individuals are more prone to develop neuroses than others (Horney 1939: 168–82). In so doing, Horney states her preference for an interpretation of anxiety as 'one of the indicators showing that something is seriously wrong with the conditions under which people live' (ibid.: 179). Accordingly, she distances herself from a conception of anxiety as a 'trait' of personality or as an experience which may be explained with exclusive reference to the vulnerabilities and weaknesses of isolated individuals. Similarly, May argues that any attempt to understand anxiety as a product of childhood experiences or as a psychosomatic disorder is incomplete unless there is a concerted effort to link the problems of psychology to a conception of the historical development of our cultural experience of the world (May 1977: 174–7). Moreover, he looks towards a sociological analysis of the changing structure of modern societies to provide him with a means of identifying the types of occasions where we are most likely to be made vulnerable to anxiety. On this basis it may be possible to chart the prevalence of anxiety as a likely consequence of the socio-economic and cultural contexts in which we find ourselves (ibid.: 171–203 and 231–9).

## The sociological discourse on anxiety

Where psychologists and psychiatrists have largely been concerned to explain the behavioural, physiological and cognitive mechanisms through which individuals acquire varieties of emotional experience, sociologists have been more interested in identifying our thoughts and feelings as a product of social structures and cultural conditions (Thoits 1995b). As far as the study of anxiety is concerned, sociologists offer ways of theorising this condition as a consequence of the social organisation, political economy and cultural values of the historical period in which we have come to identify ourselves as 'modern' people. The 'sociological imagination' may provide us with a means of self-consciously reflecting upon the ways in which the experience of anxiety is systematically reproduced as a consequence of our historical location within social structures and cultural processes which dispose us to feel, think and act in distinctively modern ways (Mills 1959: 3–24). Furthermore, where theories are applied and put to the test within the context of empirical research, sociologists have also documented the social distribution of the individual attitudes, types of relationships, economic opportunities and religious or political affiliations which are conceived as being among the main causes of anxiety. Accordingly, at the same time as sociologists have been devoted to explaining the ways in which our experience of the world is determined by our position within a distinctive social environment, they may also enable us to identify those groups and individuals who are liable to be made most vulnerable to anxiety as a consequence of their socio-economic status, the quality of their personal relationships and their levels of commitment towards the dominant cultural values of our times.

In what remains of this chapter I shall note some of the dominant theoretical themes which have come to be associated with sociological debates concerning the extent to which the social organisation of modernity is liable to make individuals prone to feel anxiously concerned about the quality of their lives. In Chapters 2 and 3 I shall concentrate in more detail upon the social distribution of the factors which are understood to make us more or less vulnerable to being in this condition. Accordingly, I am now interested to note some of the theoretical arguments and assumptions which, while being used to explain social patterns of anxiety in contemporary societies, have also served to inspire the empirical investigation of the social occasions in which we are most likely to be burdened by the sense of meaninglessness and feelings of powerlessness which comprise the subjective experience of being in anxiety.

## Individualisation

Almost all social theorists have recognised a process of individualisation as one of the most distinctive characteristics of social life under conditions of modernity. Accordingly, we are held to be living in a form of social organisation which disposes us to realise our individuality in a manner which is peculiar to the development of capitalist labour relations, the demographic shift from the country to the city and the rise of the democratic nation state. Of course, there is a sense in which people have always known themselves as individuals insofar as being in society with others endows us with a sense of personal identity and purpose; people in society always have their own social roles and obligations to perform. However, the modern experience of work and family life, combined with the opportunity to consume an historically unprecedented number of cultural goods, are widely understood to involve us in a distinctive quality of life where we are made to be increasingly aware of the peculiarity of our individual sense of identity as well as the social and historical contingency of our adopted lifestyles.

For example, industrialisation was accompanied by a rapid increase in the division of labour in society whereby it became possible for individuals to specialise in occupational activities which were unknown to those living in the agrarian communities of pre-modern societies. Anthony Giddens estimates that where there used to be no more than twenty or thirty 'traditional' trades or crafts, in modern industrial economies there are possibly more than 20,000 distinct forms of employment (Giddens 1989: 482–3). Accordingly, Emile Durkheim maintains that where there is a far greater variety of occupational types then we shall find that 'each individual is more and more acquiring his own way of thinking and acting' as a consequence of spending their working hours engaged in activities which are liable to be quite different to those of the majority of other people in society (Durkheim 1964: 137).

Moreover, with greater geographical as well as social mobility, and in particular as a consequence of the impact of feminism upon our culture, the ways in which we may experience patterns of family life have certainly become more varied and complex (Pahl 1995: 4–12). We are living in a culture where there is a great diversity of family values and the proportion of the population who are prepared to get married and subscribe to the 'orthodox' arrangement of woman as 'housewife' and man as 'breadwinner' is in marked decline (Haskey 1995). A greater onus is now placed upon individuals to work at establishing their own personal rules of conduct for their relations of intimacy, and where people engage in the practice of serial monogamy they may find that these need to be amended each time they enter into a new relationship (Giddens 1992; Beck and Beck-Gernsheim 1995).

Indeed, more generally, when it comes to organising our private lives, the globalisation of the capitalist economy ensures that we now have access to an unprecedented range of cultural goods for realising our individual passions, interests and consumer desires. So long as the financial means are available, individuals have historically unique opportunities for expressing themselves aesthetically and may buy into a great variety of cultural experiences which have only become available to us since the development of mass communication media and modern transportation networks. Aside from the fact that we are now liable to encounter a greater variety of symbolic forms of culture for exploring our inner selves and expressing our personal ideas and feelings (Thompson

1995: 207–34), perhaps more than ever before, we are in a position to recognise the historical and social contingency of our individual consciousness of the world as well as the peculiarity of our 'local' interests when contextualised in global perspective (Meyrowitz 1985; Robertson 1992).

These are just some of the factors which are thought to have brought about a profound transformation in the ways in which we experience the meaning of our place in the world, as well as our social relationships towards others and ourselves. Social conditions of modernity are understood to make us negotiate our passage through life across a wide range of different social environments and cultural contexts which require us to be permanently adaptable to the fact that our immediate surroundings and the quality of our social relationships are open to change. Accordingly, writers such as Zygmunt Bauman are inclined to argue that 'modern developments forced men and women into the condition of individuals' insofar as they 'found their lives fragmented, split into many loosely related aims and functions, each to be pursued in a different context and according to different pragmatics' (Bauman 1993: 6).

A special emphasis is placed upon the extent to which, when compared to people living in the so-called 'traditional' societies of the Middle Ages, modern individuals have a greater freedom, or rather, they are put under a greater social pressure, to decide who they shall be, how they shall live and what they shall do. In the words of Anthony Giddens: 'we have no choice but to choose how to be and how to act' (Giddens 1994a: 75). Where such 'freedom' of choice is widely understood to have given rise to the development of modern forms of rationality, the democratisation of politics and the social ethics of the rights of the individual, it has also been recognised as the source of deep feelings of insecurity which have left many people struggling to establish a sufficiently coherent (moral) meaning for their lives (Macintyre 1985; 1988; Taylor 1989). For example, Erich Fromm understands the development of modern processes of individuation to have a dialectical character: on the one hand, we have acquired a technological mastery of nature, greater powers of reason and the 'self-strength' to determine the course of our own fate, but on the other hand we are also made vulnerable to a growing sense of isolation which 'has the quality of desolation and creates an intense anxiety and insecurity' (Fromm 1942: 25). At the same time as individuals have acquired a greater freedom to arbitrate upon the meaning and direction of their lives, he suggests that, given the economic context and cultural situation in which they find themselves, most people are liable to encounter this as an 'unbearable burden' which produces a terrible 'feeling of individual insignificance and powerlessness' (ibid.: 26–32).

Indeed, the work of Erich Fromm represents one of the most consistent attempts to link the modern experience of anxiety to the process of individual-isation (Fromm 1942). Not only does he attempt to explain the historical development of the economic and cultural conditions which provide for the emergence of modern individualism, but further, he is concerned to advance a critical theory which explains why people living in industrial capitalist societies are liable to develop a 'character structure' which makes them particularly vul-nerable to anxiety. Fromm characterises the dominant experience of our individuality as one where we are most likely to be terrorised by the freedom to decide how to think and act for ourselves, moreover, he is inclined to explain this as a consequence of being denied the proper cultural resources and quality of social relationships which may enable us to realise the fullness of our human-ity in loving communion with others (Fromm 1995). With reference to Marx's theory of alienation, he argues that the drudgery and dull compulsion of work under conditions of industrial capitalism are liable to deny us our self-esteem and rob us of our self-confidence. Furthermore, he understands the competitive individualism which serves the economic dynamics of capitalist societies to impose a 'spirit of indifference' and calculating instrumentality upon the qual-ity of our social relationships whereby we are made to feel isolated with the impression that we have no value save that of being a commodity in the mar-ketplace (Fromm 1942: 102–3).

More recently, Anthony Giddens (1990; 1991; 1994a) and Ulrich Beck (1992; 1994; Beck and Beck-Gernsheim 1996) have argued that the process of individualisation has accelerated to the point where large numbers of people are becoming particularly vulnerable to an anxiety of self-identity and purpose. They maintain that where the earlier stages of industrialisation involved new ways of experiencing and realising our individuality, nevertheless, so long as there was a rigid class structure, fixed (patriarchal) gender relations as well as the possibility of acquiring a 'job for life', then people were still able to main-tain a relatively coherent sense of who they were, how they should live and what they should do. By contrast, in the closing decades of the twentieth century the 'flexibilisation' of employment, the increasing influence of feminism, the demise of the nuclear family, the extension of education as well as the prolifer-ation of mass media are all considered to have contributed towards a growing sense of disorientation in face of the fact that nothing is immutable, there are no permanent alliances and no eternal verities; more than ever before the future appears to be riven with uncertainty. In this context, Anthony Giddens suggests that where individuals encounter 'an external environment full of changes' then they will most probably become 'obsessively preoccupied with apprehension of possible risks to [their] existence, and paralysed in terms of practical action'

(Giddens 1991: 53). As a consequence they are likely to be anxiously concerned about the meaning of self-identity as well as their ability to maintain control over the course of their preferred 'lifestyle' options (ibid.: 70–108). Similarly, Ulrich Beck argues that where life in an age of 'reflexive modernisation' (Beck *et al*. 1994) is losing its 'self-evident quality', and where work and relations of intimacy are less likely to be experienced as matters of routine, then individuals are more likely to become worn out with being made to find answers to the question: 'who am I and what do I want?' (Beck and Beck-Gernsheim 1996: 31). Moreover, he also understands such conditions to make people particularly prone to experience bouts of existential anxiety (Beck 1994: 46).

The above represent just a few of the instances where writers have identified new possibilities for realising our individuality as a principal cause of anxiety in modern societies. It is important to bear in mind that the process of individualisation is one of the most heavily theorised concepts in Western sociology and considerable controversy remains as to how one should assess its overall impact upon the dominant modes of experiencing self and society under conditions of modernity. As far as the purposes of this study are concerned, I would simply draw attention to the assumption that the more we find ourselves to be living in a period of rapid social change, the more likely it is that we shall be made to be preoccupied with the possibility of maintaining a coherent sense of self-identity in face of the unpredictability of our surroundings and the absence of clear guidelines for living through the unfamiliar contexts in which we find ourselves (Giddens 1991). Moreover, it is understood that the more people find that they cannot rely upon the inviolability of established codes of rationality, the more they will discover themselves to be in a position of having to negotiate the meaning of moral rules and the difficulty of knowing how to live and what to do (Bauman 1993). In particular, where we are all party to quite different experiences of work and family life, most sociologists hold to the view that we are liable to become increasingly self-conscious of our individuality in accordance with the fact that we each have our own peculiar roles to perform, both in the context of our paid employment as well as in the home. Indeed, there are those who suspect that where people are becoming increasingly preoccupied with job insecurity and the shifting value of their relations of emotional dependency, then the social pressure towards individualisation is liable to increase as they are forced to become more reflexively oriented to the inevitability of change at work as well as in the context of the intimate relations of their private lives (Furlong and Cartmel 1997: 27–52).

Where the freedom to self-realisation is widely recognised as one of the most cherished values of modern times, writers such as Karen Horney and

Erich Fromm would alert us to the fact that the social and cultural conditions which give rise to the process of individualisation also leave large numbers of people feeling isolated and insecure with the conviction that they are being denied the opportunity to fulfil their ambitions and develop their individual potentialities. Where the majority of those living under conditions of modernity are more free to decide who they shall be and how they shall live, for many, such freedoms are encountered more as a form of oppression than a passage towards a higher meaning and purpose. Fromm emphasises that 'freedom from' the authority of tradition, the adversities of nature and the ties of community does not imply that we have attained the 'freedom to' develop our potentiality towards a full expression of our humanity (Fromm 1942: 26–31). The material conditions, cultural resources and forms of association which dispose us to encounter and know ourselves as distinct individuals, are also liable to lead us into anxiety insofar as they are all too commonly experienced as being insufficient for us to realise the fullness of our individuality. Moreover, in this context, it appears that the majority of individuals will only encounter their 'freedom' in accordance with the extent they are made to recognise themselves to be living in a social context which denies them the power and ability to withstand the threatening uncertainty of their predicament.

## The loss of community and tradition

Where social conditions of modernity are held to involve us in distinctively new ways of experiencing and realising our individuality, they are also understood to erode the ties of community and undermine the authority of tradition. From the nineteenth century to the present day, sociologists have commonly sought to analyse the character and structure of modern societies in terms of the juxtaposition between an ideal representation of life in traditional rural communities as opposed to the experience of society which emerges in the wake of industrialisation, the development of a capitalist mode of production and the rise of the metropolitan lifestyle (Nisbet 1966: 47–106). The process of individualisation is widely understood to take place in accordance with the demise of 'traditional' beliefs and values as well as the dissolution of communal modes of social organisation.

In this context, the development of the right to free speech and the toleration of religious diversity is conceived as the positive outcome of the declining influence of the Church in the affairs of public life and the triumph of a sceptical attitude which undermined the authority of religious leaders to dictate matters of truth. Moreover, the democratisation of politics, the language of civil liberties and the ethical doctrine of the rights of the individual are understood to hold no place in a social order where the privilege and status of each individual are fixed at birth and it is a mortal sin to question the authority of those (men) whose right to rule has been established as a matter of divine decree. Indeed, it is widely recognised that the emergence of 'the individual' upon the stage of Western history could only take place when we acquired a greater technological capacity to control the violence of nature and protect ourselves against the age-old hazards of famine and disease; the strong social solidarity of communal ties was in large part a necessary response to the fact that people were geographically bound to live in a hostile environment where the quality of life was most likely to be 'poor, nasty, brutish and short' (Hobbes). The cultivation of our sense of individuality rested upon the extent to which we were able to free ourselves from the social demands of communal life whereby it became possible to devote our time and energies to the development of our intellect so as to acquire the means to *self*-expression.

Nevertheless, the social life of traditional communities, at least in terms of its ideal representation within the discourse of Western social science, has often been evoked in the context of nostalgic references to a period of history in which people are thought to have been considerably less anxious about their position in society and the meaning of their lives. One of the reasons for this is to be found in the assumption that, insofar as the majority of people were not inclined (or rather, were denied the opportunity) to doubt the authority of the Church to guard 'the truth' about the natural order of the cosmos, they were also far less likely to be troubled with the kinds of 'fundamental existential questions' which have become a popular source of discontent among the denizens of modernity (Giddens 1991: 47–55). For example, Anthony Giddens maintains that the stabilising force of tradition in pre-modern societies afforded higher levels of 'ontological security' whereby people were disposed to feel more 'at home' in the world; it provided them with a clear sense of who they were and how things should be done. He explains:

> Tradition has the hold it does . . . because its moral character offers a measure of ontological security to those who adhere to it. Its psychic underpinnings are affective. There are ordinarily deep emotional investments in tradition, although these are indirect rather than direct; they come from the mechanisms of anxiety-control that traditional modes of actions and belief provide.
>
> (Giddens 1994a: 65–6)

Moreover, the forms of social organisation through which traditions are preserved and bestowed with their legislative authority are conceived as having afforded a quality of life in which people were liable to be made to feel more secure in relation to their place in the world and where they had a clearer sense of moral purpose within the emotional warmth of community.

Following Ferdinand Tonnies' typology of *Gemeinschaft* and *Gesellschaft* social relations, sociologists have often been inclined to identify the experience of living in pre-modern communities as being characterised by 'a high degree of personal intimacy, emotional depth, moral commitment, social cohesion and continuity in time' (Nisbet 1966: 47). *Gemeinschaft* relationships tend to be built around the close ties of family, neighbourhood and friendship, and as such, are considered to involve us in an experience of mutual affirmation, trust and understanding which is liable to protect us from feeling isolated and without a clear sense of self-identity. By contrast, the *Gesellschaft* relationships which characterise the social life of industrial capitalist societies are typically understood to involve 'a high degree of individualism, impersonality [and] contractualism' (ibid.: 74) whereby everyone becomes vulnerable to the feeling of loneliness and 'there exists a condition of tension against all others' (Tonnies, cited in Nisbet 1966: 76). On this view, where our lives are increasingly given over to the calculating rationality and economic individualism of *Gesellschaft* society, then we shall find ourselves more vulnerable to anxiety as a consequence of being deprived of a proper context for expressing our emotions and for sharing in the psychological intimacy of community. Without close confiding relationships and the emotional support which they provide, it is commonly agreed that, outside the ties of community, we are less able to cope with the stress of uncertainty and the threat of danger (Mirowsky and Ross 1986: 33–5).

It remains a matter of considerable controversy as to whether it is right to consider the people who lived in pre-modern traditional communities as being less prone to anxiety than the denizens of contemporary modern societies. For example, Ray Pahl (1995: 156–65) argues that such a representation of the past should be suspect on the grounds that it amounts to a form of 'golden-ageism' which, for the purpose of scoring political points or mounting moral crusades, rewrites history with a wilful ignorance of the available evidence which suggests that people have consistently struggled to cope with feelings of insecurity and have always been susceptible to the conviction that they face a future of hazardous uncertainty (at least insofar as it concerns their personal health, safety and well-being). Accordingly, he is inclined to argue that although it is undoubtedly the case that the common experience of culture, economy and society within the industrial landscape of the modern city is distinctively different from that of the traditional rural community, it is doubtful as to whether we are liable to feel any more distressed by one setting as opposed to the other.

Certainly, insofar as humanity has always been vulnerable to pain and suffering, then there is no shortage of evidence to suggest that people have consistently been burdened by the thought that they may be facing a future of acute tragedy and misery. Those who look back with romantic nostalgia towards a past where, allegedly, everyone felt more secure about their place in the world, perhaps all too easily forget that, prior to modernity, the material poverty and appalling physical health of the majority of people were a source of great anguish and discomfort. Moreover, where the irrefutable 'truths' of traditional forms of religious belief may have provided for a greater sense of 'ontological security', more often than not these left people with the firm conviction that their fate was governed by powerful supernatural forces, which without warning could bring God's judgement down upon their lives and visit them with terrible disaster. For example, in his classic study of life in a feudal society, Marc Bloch reminds us that if people managed to survive the high levels of infant mortality, then they most likely faced a (short) lifetime of constant physical suffering and fearful uncertainty. In feudal society, the presence of death was always close at hand. He writes:

> Among so many premature deaths, a large number were due to the great epidemics which descended frequently upon a humanity ill-equipped to combat them; among the poor another cause was famine. Added to the constant acts of violence these disasters gave life a quality of perpetual insecurity. This was probably one of the principal reasons for the emotional instability so characteristic of the feudal era . . . Finally we must not leave out of account the effects of an astonishing sensibility to what were believed to be supernatural manifestations. It made people's minds constantly and almost morbidly attentive to all manner of signs, dreams, or hallucinations . . . These men [were] subjected both externally and internally to so many ungovernable forces.
>
> (Bloch 1961: 73)

Nevertheless, for the sake of circumspection, I would raise a couple of points which may be used to suggest that, while people have always suffered and worried about their lives, this does not necessarily imply that they have always been prone to experience their misery as 'anxiety'. In the first place, one may take the development of a specific language of anxiety and the popularisation of the term itself, as an indication that modern people have acquired a distinctively new quality of feeling in their lives which is quite different to that of other periods of Western history. For example, both Raymond Williams (1958; 1961) and Charles Taylor (1989: 368–90) are inclined to argue that where societies undergo periods of rapid cultural change and people seek to develop new languages for expressing the differences in their experience of the world, then this may also imply a transformation within their 'felt sense of the quality of life' (Williams 1961: 61). Accordingly, one might speculate that where it is only in the last century that large numbers of people have begun to explicitly account for their symptoms of psychological distress in terms of a 'problem of anxiety' (May 1977: 3–19), then they may also be encountering a mode of feeling which is peculiar to the experience of life in contemporary modern societies.

Second, if we accept Freud's contention that a considerable part of the problem of anxiety is connected with the extent to which we are inclined to repress our instinctual drives and emotional impulses (Freud 1979: 244, 262–4), then there may be cause to suspect that people living in 'traditional' rural communities were less likely to be burdened with the specific affects of anxiety. Both Marc Bloch (1961) and Emmanuel Le Roy Ladurie (1978: 139) maintain that during the Middle Ages, people were much more prone to emotionalism. Indeed, Bloch notes that in comparison to modern times, those who lived in the age of pre-modernity seemed to be far more open with their expressions of rage and despair and were liable to give way to 'sudden revulsions of feeling' (Bloch 1961: 73). Accordingly, insofar as the moral and social conventions of feudal society did not require people to repress their emotions, one might suggest that while people felt greatly distressed by the condition of their lives, nevertheless, they may still have been less vulnerable to anxiety.

Of course, among other things, the validity of such points can only be assessed in relation to one's preferred conception of 'the problem of anxiety'. Moreover, there are many more historical and analytical factors which one may take into consideration when venturing to comment upon the differences between other ages and our own. As far as this study is concerned, I do not wish to become further embroiled in the problem of accounting for the general modes of thought and feeling which are held to characterise the different stages of history through which we have passed. However, I consider it important to highlight the extent to which such discourses have served as a major focus for debates concerning the social value of 'community' and 'tradition'.

The idea of 'community' and the alleged content of 'tradition' may well be no more than a fanciful invention of modern times, however, it is by evoking these terms that writers across the disciplines of the humanities and social sciences have ventured to define the existential condition of modern men and women and analyse their psychological complaints. The perceived breakdown, or rather, poverty of community, as experienced most obviously within the context of family relations, is understood to be a major contributory factor towards the anxious condition of modern societies. Certainly, there is a significant amount of empirical research to suggest that our capacity to cope with the stress of life is closely associated with the quality of our social ties and emotional commitments towards our family and friends (Brown and Harris 1978; Hughes and Gove 1981; Lazarus and Folkman 1984: 243–51; Mirowsky and Ross 1986: 33–5). Moreover, the extent to which the declining influence of 'traditional' forms of belief is in some way connected to the modern 'anxiety of emptiness and meaninglessness' (Tillich 1952: 52–8) remains as one of the most hotly contested debates within the philosophical discourse of modernity. Indeed, it is largely in this literary context that writers have recognised the cultural origins of the anxieties which arise in connection with the question: 'What shall we do and how shall we live?' (Weber 1948: 129–56).

## The experience of work and employment

Finally, I would emphasise the extent to which sociologists have identified the modern experience of work and employment as possibly the most significant factor within the development of social conditions and forms of culture which dispose us towards anxiety. The economic organisation of capitalist societies and the transformation of work which takes place under the drive towards modernisation are conceived to have been a major cause of the breakdown of 'traditional' forms of communal association. Moreover, it is particularly with reference to the social value of paid employment, and the quality of our social relationships at work, that sociologists have analysed the impact of individualisation upon the collective psyche of those who live under conditions of modernity.

Eric Fromm maintains that more than anything else, it was the introduction of a capitalist work ethic within the world of medieval commerce which 'destroyed [its social system] and with it the stability and relative security it had offered the individual' (Fromm 1942: 49–50). Accordingly, social status was gradually removed from the fixed ties of blood and tradition, and rather, came to be more closely associated with the level of one's success in the marketplace. Where previously work was experienced purely as a matter of sustaining one's livelihood and fulfilling one's seigneurial duties, with the advent of capitalist labour relations it acquired a new significance as the means to take control of one's destiny so as to attain personal prestige and social recognition. Moreover, in this context, a drive to maximise efficiency, the introduction of time-keeping, and the relentless pursuit of profit are held not only to have had a dramatic impact upon people's attitudes towards their working environment, but also upon their overall outlook upon life. Where on the one hand, work as paid employment acquired a greater importance as a source of individual self-identity, insofar as the quality of our social relationships in every sphere of activity was liable to come under the influence of a culture of competitive individualism, then Fromm maintains that 'a new spirit of restlessness' and cold indifference began to pervade the experience of day-to-day life (ibid.: 49–53 and 102–3) .

Where our 'freedom to' self-realisation and social recognition is understood to have been achieved according to the development of a capitalist economy and society, then sociologists have consistently alerted us to the fact that, while the modern experience of work and employment may provide for an historically unprecedented opportunity to realise our individuality, it also appears to have burdened us with a heightened sense of isolation, as well as the conviction that our destiny remains unfulfilled insofar as we are denied proper access to the material resources for pursuing our personal ambitions. Accordingly, where large numbers of people are held to be dissatisfied with the sense of worth and achievement which they may attain within the context of paid employment, then the meaning of work is understood to be a source of great frustration which is liable to make them anxiously concerned for their individual fulfilment and self-esteem (Locke and Taylor 1991). Moreover, where people are liable to suffer from unemployment or job insecurity, more often than not they are forced to contend not only with a loss of personal prestige, but also with the distress of material and social deprivation.

As I have already noted, both Rollo May (1977: 171–203) and Karen Horney (1937: 281–90) place a special emphasis upon the extent to which a culture of economic individualism not only militates against the experience of community but also burdens us with a criterion of success which we find ourselves constantly struggling to control to our benefit and purpose. More recently, Ray Pahl has argued that the theories of these writers are particularly relevant for explaining how the development of more 'flexible' patterns of employment and increasing levels of job insecurity are liable to increase the incidence of anxiety among the middle classes in Western societies. He notes that where in the middle decades of the twentieth century, the professional and managerial classes were largely protected from the threat of unemployment, it now appears that the fear of redundancy is rife among the most well-educated and materially affluent members of British and American society (Pahl 1995: 166–70). Accordingly, he maintains that these groups are more prone to develop the kinds of 'neurotic' personality traits described by Horney in her analysis of the psychology of competitiveness in modern societies (Horney 1937; 1950). Following May (1977: 358–9), Pahl suggests that insofar as middle-class professionals are likely to hold the strongest commitments to the cultural value of competitive individualism, then where they are made increasingly vulnerable to the threat of unemployment and downward social mobility, they are most liable to be made vulnerable to anxiety as a consequence of being unable to identify themselves (and be identified by others) as a 'success' at work (Pahl 1995: 166–80).

The logic of such a premise may be taken to imply that since the working classes tend to view their place of employment in more instrumental terms, as purely a source of income, then they are not so likely to be anxiously preoccupied with the meaning of their social status at work (Locke and Taylor 1991: 140–1). However, it is important to emphasise the extent to which the material and cultural circumstances of these social groups do not always afford them the luxury of such a preoccupation; there are many more immediate work-related problems for them to be anxiously concerned about. In the first place, the lower socio-economic groups in society are still burdened with the highest rates of unemployment and when made unemployed their loss of income is more likely to leave them in a state of material and social deprivation which places them at a greater risk of damage to their physical and mental health (Fryer 1995; Bartley *et al.* 1999). Second, their working and domestic environments tend to be more dangerous and these groups tend to suffer more accidents and are more likely to be the victims of violent crime (Wilkinson *et al.* 1998). Third, the stress of work and the poverty of their living conditions are most probably a major contributive factor to the higher rates of divorce and family breakdown among the lower classes. Certainly, women in classes IV and V are still likely to be diagnosed as suffering from more anxiety and depressive disorders than women in classes I and II (Acheson 1998: 16). Moreover, the levels of drug and alcohol dependence, which are considered to be a principal means by which people struggle to cope with their symptoms of distress and anxiety, are far greater among working-class men. Indeed, the rate of suicide for those in class V is almost four times higher than for those in classes I and II (Acheson 1998: 12) and it is even greater among the unemployed (Charlton *et al.* 1993).

Accordingly, it appears that different socio-economic groups are liable to encounter their anxieties in connection with contrasting types of social problems and threats to their personal health and security. While the anxiety of the middle classes is for the most part conceived to be related to their sense of self-esteem and the stress of competition in the workplace, they are less likely to suffer the anguish of material deprivation and do not appear to be so vulnerable to stress-related illnesses and disease. By contrast, where they are sometimes represented as not being so preoccupied with the meaning of their work, the anxiety of the working classes appears to be more closely related to the threat of violence and physical harm, the risk of family breakdown, the distress of material deprivation and a higher risk of unemployment. In both instances, the experience of work and employment is conceived to be a major source of anxiety in contemporary societies. Moreover, insofar as sociologists may point towards solutions to anxiety, or rather, advise us as to how we might better cope with its disruptive impacts upon our lives, then it is most likely that they will devote the large part of their analysis to the meaning and necessity of work. Indeed, insofar as we may be freed from the 'stress of necessity', Freud himself recognised the modern preoccupation with work as not only a major determining factor in the development of Western civilisation, but also as a principal means towards the possibility of attaining mental health (Freud 1985: 267–8).

## A sociological conception of anxiety

Within the context of sociology, being vulnerable to the 'problem of anxiety' is conceived not so much as a consequence of individuals having something 'wrong' with them, but rather, as the result of social antagonisms and cultural contradictions which comprise their common experiences of day-to-day life. Sociologists are inclined to recognise the prevalence of anxiety as a sign that people are being denied the proper social conditions for keeping themselves in good health, rather than privileging an interpretation of anxiety which locates its origins within the personality 'traits' of the individual. Accordingly, David Smail suggests that we should hold to the conviction that:

> Our subjective experience of the world tells us the truth about it, even if the language it has to do so is cast in forms we have come to see as symptoms. We live in anxiety, fear and dread because these constitute a proper response to the nature of our social world.
>
> (Smail 1984: 98)

I have noted some of the main theoretical themes which, at the level of socio-logical discourse, have been used to analyse the social and cultural conditions which are understood to make people vulnerable to develop those symptoms of psychological emotional and physiological distress which we have come to refer to as 'anxiety'. Of course, these are by no means adequate to equip us with a complete account of 'the nature of our social world', rather, they merely provide a simplified abstraction of a selective range of factors which we may consider to be implicated within the anxious condition of modern societies. Nevertheless, for the purposes of this study it is hoped that they are sufficiently relevant to be used as a means of analysing some of the sociological indicators of anxiety which are to be explored in more detail in the following chapter. Moreover, in this context I have already introduced some of the critical themes which will be used for evaluating the contention that we are becoming more anxious in accordance with the extent to which we are made more 'risk conscious'.

It is particularly with this end purpose in mind that I have been concerned to focus upon the problem of defining anxiety. While presenting the reader with a selective account of the influence of cultural conditions upon the psychological and bodily components of anxiety, I have also sought to emphasise the extent to which the subjective experience of this condition may be understood to impose itself upon our consciousness as a problem of culture. Accordingly, I have offered a definition of anxiety which highlights some of the ways in which this experience takes place in the context of a struggle for (self-)definition and a search for meaning. Anxiety is a problem of culture insofar as it impresses upon us a desperate desire to equip ourselves with a means of 'seeing' our way through a situation of foreboding obscurity so as to cast light upon methods of avoiding or confronting a threatening danger.

In this context, the trauma of anxiety is understood to function as a means whereby we might attain a clearer conception of the fearful situations in which we find ourselves. While making itself known to all, anxiety always keeps us under the conviction that its precise meaning and purpose remain outside our knowledge, and thereby we are driven to find a sufficient means of identifying 'the truth' of our predicament. Indeed, this is why Søren Kierkegaard is inclined to recognise the experience of anxiety, not only as a reaction to the threat of danger, but also as a source of spiritual education (Kierkegaard 1980: 155–62). Similarly, while Rollo May devotes the large part of his analysis to the psychological distress of anxiety, he would also alert us to its creative purpose as a cause of intellectual invention and artistic inspiration (May 1977: 384–93). Thus, one might recognise the condition of anxiety not only as a sign of cultural loss and deprivation, but also (insofar as we may remain distressed by the trauma of this experience), as a potential source of cultural creativity and renewal.

# A SOCIOLOGICAL CONCEPTION OF THE PROBLEM OF ANXIETY

Ultimately, I propose that it is by analysing the complex associations between culture, knowledge, fear and anxiety that we might reach a critical vantage point for evaluating the social and political significance of the 'risk debate' in contemporary Western societies. In this chapter I have simply attempted to introduce the reader to a range of complex issues involved within the study of anxiety. In particular, I have been concerned to highlight some of the distinctive analytical components of a sociological conception of the problem of anxiety. While in this context I have focused for the most part upon the possibility of conceptualising anxiety as a product of social conditions and cultural predispositions, I would also add that I believe it is important for sociologists to consider the specific emotional, cognitive and behavioural components of the individual experience of day-to-day life. I am writing under the conviction that a critical reflection upon the idea of social structure also requires us to engage in the attempt to demonstrate its impacts upon the mentalities and emotions of individuals in the 'real' world. For sociology to deliver 'the promise' of helping us to understand ourselves 'as minute points in the intersections of biography and history within society' (Mills 1959: 7), it needs to remain alert and relevant to the particular ways in which we become self-consciously aware of our personal struggles and confusions. With these ambitions in mind, I now turn to consider the possibility of establishing sociologically 'objective' indicators of the prevalence and levels of anxiety in contemporary British society.

# 2

---

# Social indicators of anxiety

It is now a matter of sociological common sense to identify ourselves as living through a period of acute insecurity and high anxiety. Indeed, many would recognise the condition of anxiety as the most prominent component of the prevailing cultural consciousness of modern times (Kroker and Cook 1988; Giddens 1991: i–vii; Beck 1992: 49; Pahl 1995; Dunant and Porter 1996; Furedi 1997; Vail *et al.* 1999). As a matter of cultural commentary the brute facts of anxiety appear to be almost beyond dispute. Where the mass media supply us with a relentless flow of information on alarming social problems and hazardous events, one may well presume that the majority of people are readily convinced that levels of anxiety surrounding the security of our world are now more pronounced than ever before. However, while we might all possess good reasons to be anxious, these do not necessarily translate into *feelings* of anxiety (Wilkinson 1999). While 'anxiety' may well be recognised as a theme which is most consonant with the cultural narrative of late modernity, it is quite another thing to identify public discourses on anxiety as a clear indication of the extent to which people actually feel distressed by the quality of their lives. Our social interactions with popular discourses on the anxieties of modern societies need not make us prone to experience this condition for ourselves.

In this chapter I am concerned to explore the extent to which it may be possible to identify those social groups which are most vulnerable to experience the emotional distress of being in anxiety. What evidence can we look to in order to establish the extent to which people actually *feel* burdened by the problems which anxiety brings to their lives? Is it possible to use empirical research as a means of assessing the allegation that large sections of the populations of advanced industrial nations are currently preoccupied with the task of coping with acute levels of distress? Moreover, can anxiety be quantified so that we may provide an accurate measurement of the extent to which it disrupts the lives of modern people? Indeed, may we reach any definitive conclusions as to who has the most anxiety and how far can we agree upon the social factors which are responsible for making them feel this way?

Throughout my discussion I draw critical attention to the interpretive decisions that researchers make in order to establish the presence and prevalence of anxiety among different sectors of the population. We can never actually enter into another person's feelings; feelings of anxiety may only be experienced uniquely as our own. When inquiring into the proper identity of another's feelings we are presented with the task of making a selective interpretation of the meanings of the physiological reactions and symbolic forms of culture which are used to express outwardly the contents of their inner experiences of body and mind. Moreover, I am concerned to argue that when venturing to recognise the presence of anxiety in other people we are committed to a hermeneutical process which is always open to conflicting interpretations as to the 'true' meanings of forms of communication and behaviour.

When it comes to the possibility of determining the levels of anxiety in society as a whole, I refer predominantly to the works of those concerned with revealing the prevalence of psychiatric morbidity in contemporary society. While this literature tends to be narrowly focused upon the aetiological significance of anxiety for different types of mental disorder, nevertheless, it has involved the most concerted efforts to establish the overall amount of anxiety in society as a fact of empirical research. Moreover, where researchers have ventured to correlate measurements of psychiatric morbidity with the social distribution of stressful life events and processes, then a number of writers consider us to be in a position where we can identify the 'objective' structural conditions which are most likely to arouse the experience of anxiety. Indeed, many hold to the view that empirical sociology is now in a position to identify authoritatively the 'core facts' as to the prevailing patterns of social distress in advanced industrial societies (Mirowsky and Ross 1986; Thoits 1995a; Turner *et al.* 1995).

However, while it is possible to clearly demonstrate the distressing effects of particular types of events and processes upon the lives of large numbers of people, it is quite another thing to explain why and how this takes place. Indeed, where the majority of those who comprise the social groups which display the most symptoms of psychological distress still remain remarkably 'healthy' in terms of their vulnerability to depression and anxiety disorder, then attention has turned to the problem of identifying the key variables which might be used to explain why some people are more able to cope with distressing circumstances than others (Brown *et al.* 1987). Accordingly, a growing number of researchers have come to emphasise that it is particularly in relation to the *meanings* which individuals acquire and create for the objective social conditions in which they find themselves, that we may piece together an explanation for differences in the intensity of their experiences of depression and anxiety (Brown and Harris 1989; Riessman 1989; Turner and Avison 1992; Pearlin 1991; Simon 1995; 1997).

In keeping with my emphasis upon the cultural components of the 'problem of anxiety', I am particularly concerned to highlight the theoretical and method-ological implications of the moderating force of meaning upon our vulnerability to experiences of psychological distress. I would argue that the latent 'discov-ery' of the experience of distress as moderated by the negative meanings of events in our lives may be used, not only to highlight the analytical strengths of more qualitative in-depth approaches to the study of mental health, but also to alert us to the extent to which the social distribution of anxiety is determined by cultural processes which are by no means fixed or constant. I would represent the experience of anxiety as a cultural reality which is embedded within variable and dynamic processes of social determination where there is always scope for each person to reappraise the meanings of the stressful situations in which they find themselves. On this basis, it is important to recognise the provisional char-acter of all accounts of the prevalence of anxiety at any particular time and place; in the long term, the 'core facts' about the social distribution of anxiety may always be subject to revision.

In the first section I examine the methodological task of interpreting another person's feelings as 'anxiety'. This is intended to provide the foundations for a critical review of some of the ways in which researchers attempt to measure the prevalence of anxiety throughout society as a whole. For the sake of establish-ing statistically reliable assessments of the social distribution of psychological distress, researchers are discouraged from becoming involved with the idio-syncrasies of meanings which symptoms hold for their respondents. However, when turning to consider the bearing of social conditions upon individuals' dif-ferential vulnerability to anxiety, I aim to highlight the extent to which it is *only* when we are prepared to consider the subjective meanings which people acquire and create for events in their lives that we may begin to piece together a more complete explanation for the prevalence of psychological distress among different sectors of the population. In the final section I argue that while it is possible to identify the types of social events and processes which make people vulnerable to anxiety, when we become alert to the moderating force of meaning upon our psychology we might also be in a position to recognise that their experience of anxiety is determined by cultural processes which are always open to change. Accordingly, I refer to the current transformation of British family life and new developments in the search for intimacy as examples of social contexts where it appears that researchers may have to substantially revise their understandings of the types of relationships which are most conducive to our mental health.

## To know another's feelings

There are many different forms of culture through which we may express the content of our feelings, but it is only in the last century that large numbers of people have come to explicitly refer to a portion of their emotional and psychological distress in terms of the 'problem of anxiety' (May 1977: 3–19). 'Anxiety' may well be just a modern name for an age-old feeling which is an inevitable consequence of the psychic constitution of our humanity. Accordingly, in a secular culture one might recognise the language of psychology to have replaced that of religion as the preferred means of interpreting the felt quality of our inner experience of life; when it comes to discussing matters of feeling, we now prefer to speak with deference to the authority of experts in the fields of human science rather than the (more doubtful) wisdom of those who would explain our problems in terms of our relationship towards God. However, in taking up the language of anxiety, perhaps we have not only come to explain ourselves differently, but further, we may also have begun to modify the way we feel.

Raymond Williams (1961: 63–6) suggests that each culture has its own peculiar structure of feeling. Language is but a small part of the many elements which comprise a whole way of life which, retrospectively, we may identify as belonging to a distinctive period of our cultural history. Where it is possible for us to document a change in the use of language, this may not only mark a shift of attitudes and behaviour, but also, in the 'felt sense of the quality of life' for those living in a particular time and place. Moreover, Williams contends that even where we find successive generations who speak 'the same language', we should still expect each to possess its own distinctive sense of style and expression whereby they are likely to feel somewhat differently about their lives. He argues:

> One generation may train its successor, with reasonable success, in the social character or the general pattern, but the new generation will have its own structure of feeling, which will not appear to have come 'from' anywhere . . . the new generation responds in its own ways to the unique world it is inheriting, taking up many continuities, that can be traced, and reproducing many aspects of the [prevailing social] organisation, which can be separately described, yet feeling its whole life in certain ways differently, and shaping its creative response into a new structure of feeling.
>
> (ibid.: 65)

When it comes to drawing comparisons between the feelings of generations, Williams is adamant that we can never know the full sense of the actual lived experience of people other than ourselves. Past feelings remain irrecoverable. We may use our own experiences to make speculative interpretations as to how others may have felt about their lives, but we should remain mindful of the fact that each interpretation (and subsequent reinterpretation) is highly selective and is bound to include many important omissions and distortions. Indeed, even when we look back upon our own lives, we are unlikely to remember the precise quality of our earlier experience of the world, for we never remain still; our memories of how we once were will inevitably be reduced and re-evaluated in accordance with our shifting interests and concerns. We may only lay hold to an abstract version of events from our past; and all the more so if we would speak of the past experiences of other people (ibid.: 65–6).

Similarly, Freud advises that it is 'impossible for us to feel our way' into how other people actually experience the inner quality of their lives (Freud 1985: 277). Feelings are essentially subjective. As a matter of scientific investigation, we can describe the physiological signs of feeling, however, where this is impossible, we are left with no choice but to interpret the meanings of the symbolic forms of culture which people use to outwardly express the contents of their inner experience of life. Moreover, at this point, we may always be left with questions as to whether our interpretation is correct, and further, we may still doubt whether the subjects of our investigation were able to provide a proper symbolic representation of what they were feeling at a particular time and place (ibid.: 252). Indeed, for Freud, the task of psychoanalysis is made even more complicated by the fact that there are occasions where people seem to be barely conscious of the 'true' identity of their feelings; the substantial part of the 'reality' of what we feel may well remain locked in the unconscious (ibid.: 328–9).

In the first instance 'anxiety' is simply the name we give to an unpleasant feeling. However, as Freud and many others since have been all too aware, when it comes to saying precisely what anxiety is, we soon find that 'anxiety is not so simple a matter' (Freud 1979: 288). There is still no consensus as to what types of unpleasant feeling are most appropriately interpreted as 'anxiety', and matters are made considerably more complicated by those researchers who lay emphasis upon the fact that anxiety is more than just a physiological sensation, rather, it is an experience constructed out of the meanings, values, self-images and expectations through which we relate to others and ourselves. Anxiety is not only a state of emotion, it is also a state of mind. Our vulnerability to anxiety appears to be moderated by the ways we construct meanings for the situations in which we find ourselves; anxiety is an affect of our knowledge of self and society.

For us to identify the presence of anxiety in an individual, then we are not only faced with the task of interpreting expressions of physiological behaviour and symbolic forms of culture through which they give representation to their feelings, but also with having to evaluate the experiential content of the values and beliefs which give meaning to their existence. For example, in his case studies of unmarried mothers, Rollo May seeks to establish the presence of anxiety in his respondents by making careful study of their language and facial expressions in order to note signs of inner conflicts, repressed guilt feelings and underlying fears. Where one of the women appears to 'laugh off' his suggestions as to the possible identity of her fears, he interprets this as evasive behaviour which betrays the presence of hidden feelings of conflict and hostility. In another instance, he interprets the long pauses before a respondent replies to his questions as a sign that they are being cautious in order to protect themselves against 'anxiety-creating emotional involvements' (May 1977: 339). Moreover, he maintains that the conversation of those suffering from the most severe forms of anxiety tends to display a considerable discrepancy between their ideal expectations for their lives as opposed to the 'reality' in which they are made to live. Accordingly, May's assessment of the severity of the anxiety experience involves not only an interpretation of the ways in which language and behaviour reveal 'the truth' about the content of our inner feelings, but also a judgement as to the extent to which our expectations for reality come into conflict with 'the world as it is' so that we are most likely to be left feeling disoriented, helpless and trapped (ibid.: 263–359).

Matters are made considerably more complicated by the fact that, in the practice of empirical research, it is sometimes very difficult to witness clear distinctions between the experience of anxiety as opposed to the many other types of unpleasant feelings which sometimes take 'noisy possession' of our consciousness (Freud 1985: 328). Where as a point of theoretical analysis one might be inclined to explain anxiety in contradistinction to other emotional states such as fear, shame and guilt, when one is faced with the task of interpreting the proper meaning of human language and behaviour in the 'real world', it is often extremely difficult to establish clear signs of one of these emotional states as being distinct from the others. For example, in the context of health psychology, Stanley Rachman notes that even when practitioners are able to draw upon a clear set of analytical criteria for making formal distinctions between the various types of phobia, anxiety disorders and states of depression, when it comes to the practice of categorising their patients' language and behaviour in these terms, then their diagnostic assessments are far from being wholly reliable. Where most are able to highlight a range of ideal–typical examples of the ways in which individuals are understood to manifest the symptoms of a particular disorder, there are many cases where it is extremely difficult to be certain that the correct meanings have been given to the complexity of outward physiological appearances and symbolic forms of expression. Certainly, practitioners should expect their professional opinions to be questioned and possibly disputed by their colleagues, not least because at the level of technical language there is no universally accepted definition of anxiety, and certainly, there is no overall consensus as to how this term should be used within the official diagnosis of mental illness (Rachman 1998: 4–7).

Where researchers have devised a clear set of heuristic principles and interpretive hypotheses for reading the presence of anxiety within the language and behaviour of their respondents, then they should anticipate having to adapt the ways these are put into practice so as to accommodate the fact that individuals are liable to respond to stressful situations in a wide variety of ways. For example, Rollo May conducts his research according to the basic assumption that being an unmarried mother and living in a women's hostel amounts to a 'crisis situation' in which they are most likely to be burdened by some kind of anxiety; however, during his interviews he discovers a wide range of individual attitudes and reactions to this predicament. In each instance, May's questions elicit different kinds of verbal and behavioural responses; while he understands some to be displaying clear signs of inner conflicts and underlying fears, others appear to successfully cope with, or adapt to, their situation so as to avoid anxiety. He refers to variables such as the ways in which the women experienced their upbringing, social status and ethnic origin in order to read a variety of different meanings into their responses to his questions. The ways in which he applies his questions and interprets the women's replies appear to be determined not only according to his understanding of what it means to be either 'black' or 'white', and 'working-class' or 'middle-class', but also by his assessment of the women's individual personality traits and their subjective sense of the 'reality' in which they find themselves. It is only after he has negotiated his way through a dense complex of interpretive decisions that he considers himself to have reached a position where he is able to rank each individual according to their vulnerability to anxiety. Moreover, he is careful to highlight the extent to which he is only able to offer a snapshot assessment of the ways in which the women appear to handle their situation at a particular time and place; he anticipates the likelihood that in the future each individual's vulnerability to anxiety will change according to the possibilities which are open to them to take different courses of action in response to the threatening situations in which they find themselves (May 1977: 320).

In what follows, I shall inquire into the possibility of using empirical research as a means of establishing social indicators for the overall prevalence of anxiety in contemporary society. Accordingly, I will attempt to move beyond the problem of discovering how an individual experiences their particular symptoms of anxiety to the point where it may be possible to pass comment upon the collective contents of the thoughts and feelings of large sections of the population as a whole. Such a project presumes that, notwithstanding the great complexity and analytical obscurity of its object of investigation, one might still be able to establish a broad overview of the general state and social distribution of anxiety in our society. Indeed, as a matter for empirical investigation, it holds to the view that one may gather reliable data for demonstrating, and possibly explaining, the link between 'public issues of social structure' such as the rate of unemployment, marriage and divorce and the experiences of anxiety which comprise the ways individuals sometimes feel about their 'personal troubles of milieu' (Mills 1959: 8).

## Measurements of anxiety

It is only since the 1980s that researchers within the field of clinical psychology have reached a working consensus on how to interpret the meanings of physiological expressions and symbolic representations of feeling so that the majority may now share an understanding of what constitutes signs of 'anxiety' (Rachman 1998: 1). Classification schemes such as *The Diagnostic and Statistical Manual of Mental Disorders* (DSM) (American Psychiatric Association 1994) and the *International Classification of Diseases* (ICD) (World Health Organization 1993b) have provided psychiatrists and psychologists with 'official' languages for specifying the diagnostic criteria for particular types of mental disorder. However, while the majority of practitioners may now be committed to using standardised lists of definitions for diagnosing the symptoms of extreme forms of emotional distress, when it comes to the practice of classifying individual behaviours and experiences in these terms, then there is still a considerable amount of controversy surrounding the reliability of clinical assessments of our psychological health.

In the first place, certain types of disorder appear to be easier to diagnose than others. For example, in research designed to test the diagnostic reliability of the *Schedule for Affective Disorders and Schizophrenia – Lifetime Anxiety Version* (SADS-LA), Salvatore Mannuzza and colleagues found that where clinicians are usually able to agree upon the symptoms which constitute signs of 'generalized anxiety', 'panic' and 'obsessive-compulsive disorders', they find it far more difficult to reach a consensus on what types of experiences and behaviours should be diagnosed as a simple 'phobia' (Mannuzza *et al.* 1989). Indeed, where it is often possible to make several diagnoses out of clinical assessments of psychiatric disorder, then this is understood to represent a serious challenge to those who aspire to make 'reliable' comparisons between separate studies of anxiety and other affective disorders (Mannuzza *et al.* 1989; Fryer *et al.* 1989). Moreover, this problem is exacerbated by the fact that, while researchers may share the same language for categorising symptoms of distress as forms of 'disorder', there are many different methods of gathering data for diagnosis. For instance, Gavin Andrews and Lorna Peters are moved to complain about the extent to which

> Individual clinicians apply their own rules about eliciting and amalgamating information, rules which may differ from those applied by other clinicians, and which may differ from occasion to occasion even with the same clinician, thus rendering clinical diagnoses unreliable.
>
> (Andrews and Peters 1999: 1)

In an attempt to promote more 'reliable' methods of gathering data on the symptoms of disorder, various structured diagnostic interview techniques such as the *Composite International Diagnostic Interview* (CIDI) (World Health

Organization 1993a), have been developed with the aim of establishing some standard criteria for assessing the quality of our mental health. In most cases, the questions on anxiety tend to be concerned with subjective assessments of types and episodes of unpleasant feelings, and in particular, a special emphasis is placed upon the extent to which individuals report having experienced a range of behaviours which are symptomatic of being in a state of acute distress. Interviewers provide a score for the number of symptoms reported in a session, and on this basis, a clinical assessment of the severity of their condition is gathered as data to be diagnosed as forms of disorder.

In this context, researchers are not required to define anxiety in relation to any detailed exploration of the meanings which symptoms hold for their informants, rather, they are primarily concerned to identify its presence in terms of a list of distressing behaviours and physiological sensations. For the most part, the questions are fully specified and are designed to elicit a simple yes/no response, for if researchers were to intervene in order to probe more deeply into the personal meanings of individual respondents' replies, then this would require them to use non-standardised techniques, which in terms of the conditions of 'reliability' are judged to compromise the possibility of making inter-study comparisons. In each instance, the onus is placed upon the respondent to offer a simple interpretation of the general state of their thoughts and feelings, while the severity of their condition is largely assessed in terms of the range and frequency of the physiological responses which comprise their experiences of distress. Accordingly, for the most part, the condition of anxiety is being conceived of as a physically debilitating problem, as opposed to an experience constructed out of the images, values and beliefs which give meaning to our lives.

For example, in the revised version of the *Clinical Interview Schedule* (CIS-R) (Lewis and Pelosi 1990), which is used by the Office of Population Censuses and Surveys as a means of inquiring into the prevalence of psychiatric morbidity in Great Britain, the section on anxiety requires interviewers to ask their respondents whether, how often and how long they had experienced heart racing or pounding, hand sweating or shaking, feeling dizzy, difficulty getting breath, butterflies in stomach, a dry mouth, nausea or feeling as though he/she wanted to vomit (Meltzer *et al.* 1994: 11). While similar forms of physiological reactions and sensations are understood to accompany an episode of 'phobia', in this schema a distinction is made between anxiety and phobia on the grounds that when the latter is experienced the informant reports that they were able to adopt some kind of avoidance behaviour in order to mitigate the effects of their distress. The *Clinical Interview Schedule* is also used to inquire into a wide range of the other anxiety-related symptoms which are understood to comprise the experience of emotional and cognitive disorder, such as 'sleep problems', 'obsessions', 'worry', 'irritability', and 'depressive ideas'. In this first instance, it is up to the respondent to interpret the content of their feelings and offer an account of their severity, while experts offer a clinical assessment of their condition according to how often they are able to recognise themselves as having experienced a select range of physiological symptoms of disorder.

For the sake of establishing some 'objective' criteria for measuring anxiety as an outwardly observable form of distress, the most 'reliable' research schemes for investigating the prevalence of psychiatric morbidity place an emphasis upon the task of counting different types of physiological reactions and behaviours so as to discourage individual researchers from getting too involved in the idiosyncrasies of meaning which these symptoms hold for their respondents. However, from the point of view of authorities such as Rollo May, who would reserve the term 'anxiety' to refer to an existential condition in which individuals struggle to come to terms with the threatening and indefinite meanings of events in their lives, then those who use structured diagnostic interviews for making assessments of our psychiatric condition may not yet be in a position to recognise the 'problem of anxiety' as the underlying cause of our distress. Indeed, May argues that it is only where we can show that distressing physiological sensations and behaviours have been 'cued off by a threat to some value that the individual holds essential to his existence as a personality' that we may venture to categorise their condition as 'anxiety' (May 1977: 205). Moreover, while Sigmund Freud acknowledges that anxiety is liable to affect our heart rate and respiratory organs, in his later essays on 'Inhibitions, Symptoms and Anxiety' (1926), the large part of his analysis focuses upon the extent to which the most distinguishing characteristics of this condition are to be found in the trauma of perceiving oneself to be facing an unknown quantity of danger (Freud 1979: 288–301). Accordingly, where a general assessment of our psychiatric condition is made largely on the evidence of physiological reactions and behaviours, then researchers may well be accused of committing themselves to interpretive decisions which go beyond the limits of what can be properly discerned from outwardly observable symptoms. Where for the sake of inter-study reliability they are made to use standardised methods of categorisation which have little regard for the peculiar ways in which individuals in society negotiate the meaning of the threatening uncertainties of their personal circumstances, then they may well be neglecting the very components of our experience which are among the most distinctive attributes of the existential condition of being *in* anxiety.

However, in this context, it is important to note that where studies are inclined to focus our attention upon physiological symptoms of distress, then they tend not to be so much concerned to advance our understanding of the 'problem of anxiety' *per se*, but rather, with the extent to which a variety of different types of unpleasant psychological states may be linked to an episode of mental and/or physical illness. While such an approach offers a range of empirical criteria for assessing the prevalence of anxiety in contemporary societies, the almost exclusive focus upon the aetiological significance of the 'physiology of anxiety' (Freud 1979: 288) leaves a large portion of the phenomenological experience of our psychology outside the domain of what is 'officially' recognised by health researchers as a problem of anxiety. Most purported measurements of anxiety have little regard for the interrelationship between anxiety, culture and meaning, rather, the majority of research schemes are simply designed to document the incidence of different forms of psychophysiological distress. Indeed, it appears that many researchers are inclined to treat 'measures of malaise, anxiety, and depression [as] interrelated and interchangeable for most purposes' (Mirowsky and Ross 1986: 25). For example, John Mirowsky and Catherine Ross work according to the premise that, in the majority of cases, those who appear to be most distressed or burdened by some kind of malaise are also most likely to be suffering from the highest levels of anxiety (ibid.). Similarly, Richard Lazarus identifies anxiety as a 'stress emotion' which is strongest among those people who perceive themselves to be poorly equipped to cope with the routine pressures and daily hassles of their world (Lazarus 1999: 58).

In the context of stress research,[1] the condition of anxiety, along with feelings of depression and a general sense of malaise, is conceived as an aetiologically significant form of distress which may be accounted for in terms of the social distribution of chronic stressors, such as a lengthy period of unemployment and economic hardship, and disruptive life-changing events, such as divorce and bereavement (Pearlin 1989: 243–6; Holmes and Rahe 1967; Ross and Mirowsky 1979; Miller and Rahe 1997). Moreover, since efforts have been made to correlate the data gathered by structured interview schedules for the measurement of mental and physical illness with the results of questionnaires designed to reveal the numbers of stressful life events and processes in respondents' lives (Pearlin 1989; Turner *et al.* 1995), then some have ventured to identify the experience of distress as a socially determined process with empirically demonstrable 'effects' upon our health (Mirowsky and Ross 1986; Aneshensel *et al.* 1991). Indeed, where researchers are now able to agree that the experience of distress is unevenly distributed throughout different sections of the population, then it may be possible for us to monitor certain types of objective social conditions and life events as manifest indicators of the prevalence of anxiety in society.

## The social distribution of anxiety as 'distress'

According to the most recent report by the Office of Population Censuses and Surveys into the prevalence of psychiatric morbidity in Great Britain, 14 per cent of adults aged 16 to 64 are currently experiencing some kind of neurotic health problem. The most common neurotic symptoms as measured by the *Clinical Interview Schedule* were fatigue (27 per cent), sleep problems (25 per cent), irritability (22 per cent) and worry (20 per cent). The most prevalent neurotic disorders, as diagnosed according to the criteria of the *International Classification of Diseases*, were mixed anxiety and depressive disorder (71/1000) followed by generalised anxiety disorder (30/1000) (Meltzer *et al.* 1994). When it comes to identifying the types of people which are most likely to be suffering from a problem of psychological disorder, there is now considerable accumulated evidence to demonstrate an association between mental health and forms of stratification such as class, gender and age. Moreover, most stress researchers understand the weight of empirical evidence to reveal the institutional organisation of our social relationships at work and in the home to have a structural bearing upon our vulnerability to anxiety-related illness and disease (Pearlin 1989; Mirowsky and Ross 1986; Aneshensel *et al.* 1991; Aneshensel 1992; Turner *et al.* 1995).

It is widely agreed that members of the lower socio-economic classes are likely to display the most symptoms of psychological distress (Kessler and Cleary 1980; Thoits 1995a: 55). In recent years a number of studies have discovered that lower income groups tend to exhibit the highest baseline levels of blood cortisol;[2] a physiological reaction which is now understood to be a key determinant in the onset of depression and recurrent episodes of severe states of anxiety (Brunner and Marmot 1999). Women in classes VI and V are more likely than those in classes I and II to be diagnosed as suffering from some kind of neurotic disorder, and levels of alcohol and drug dependency are far higher among men in lower socio-economic groups (Acheson 1998: 16). Moreover, in England and Wales, there is a clear association between social class and the rate of suicide, and current trends indicate that members of class V are far more likely than any other group to take their own lives (Drever *et al.* 1996; Marmot 1999: 4).

Such factors may be explained with reference to the fact that these people are subjected to a way of life in which they are made to experience more distressing events than those in higher socio-economic groups (Pearlin 1989: 247–7; Aneshensel 1992: 20–2). In addition to the persistent economic hardships of low income households, they are more likely to be situated in the socially deprived parts of cities which suffer from the highest rates of violent crime and environmental pollution. Manual workers are more likely to suffer lengthy periods of unemployment; an experience which is understood by the majority of health psychologists to be heavily implicated within the onset of both mental and physical illness (Aneshensel 1992: 30–1; Fryer 1995). Moreover, changes in the structure of labour markets in advanced industrial nations have resulted in these groups being more vulnerable than most to job insecurity and deteriorating working conditions; factors which are now widely understood to be among the major causes of the insecurity of contemporary societies (Wheelock 1999). According to Richard Wilkinson, it appears that a considerable portion of the chronic anxieties of lower income groups may be attributed to the fact that they are most prone to experience a sense of 'shame, inferiority and subordination' as a result of the ways in which they perceive themselves in relation to the prevailing social hierarchy (Wilkinson 1999: 260–5). Furthermore, there is growing evidence to suggest that income inequality is closely associated with a breakdown of 'civic community' whereby those at the lower end of the income scale are more likely to suffer the adverse effects of poor social relations which are lacking in emotional support (ibid.). Indeed, men and women in lower socio-economic groups are less likely to get married and/or remain in long-standing confiding/emotional relationships (Haskey 1996; Stansfield 1999). Levels of family conflict, parental separation and divorce have consistently been shown to be greatest among those groups who experience the most economic deprivation, unemployment, job insecurity and poor housing (Wadsworth 1999: 48–53).

According to the OPCS survey of psychiatric morbidity in Britain, women are almost twice as likely as men to suffer from some kind of neurotic health problem (Meltzer *et al.* 1994: 5). Moreover, the majority of mental health studies in Britain and the United States have consistently found women to exhibit the most symptoms of anxiety and depressive disorder (Mirowsky and Ross 1986; Thoits 1995a: 55). There are two main explanations for this fact. In the first place, there is a well-established tradition of research which identifies the social roles which women occupy as 'housewife' and 'child minder' to expose them to a disproportionate amount of distress (Gove 1972; Gove and Tudor 1973; Brown and Harris 1978). In this context, a particular emphasis is placed upon the negative and devalued social meanings which have become attached to women's family and occupational roles whereby they are liable to experience higher levels of 'status frustration' and are more likely to be denied the material and cultural resources for exercising control over their lives (Mirowsky and Ross 1986: Simon 1995; 1997). A second approach focuses upon the evidence which suggests that women are more likely than men to become involved in social networks where the burden of caring/emotional commitments is liable to increase their vulnerability to distress (Kessler and McLeod 1984). For example, in their study of the 'epidemiology of social stress', R. Jay Turner and colleagues found evidence to suggest that women's higher levels of distress are most likely to be aroused in connection with the disruptive events in the lives of family members and close friends. Accordingly, they argue that 'women tend to have a wider domain of social concern' whereby they are more likely to bear 'an emotional cost of caring' (Turner *et al*. 1995: 113).

However, it is important to note that the evidence which suggests that women are more prone to anxiety than men rests largely upon clinical measures of psychiatric morbidity. Where researchers have considered factors such as the rates of substance abuse and suicide, it is possible to form quite different judgements about gender differences in the social distribution of anxiety. For example, a number of researchers claim that since it appears that men may be as much as three times more likely to have an alcohol dependency and are twice as likely to be drug dependent (Meltzer *et al*. 1994), then we should be far more cautious when it comes to concluding that women are more distressed than men (Pearlin 1989: 253; Aneshensel *et al*. 1991). Peggy Thoits suggests that if women's depressive symptoms and men's alcohol abuse are viewed as alternative types of reaction to distress, then researchers should be more concerned to investigate gender differences in the ways in which people are socialised to express and cope with their experiences of distress (Thoits 1995a: 56). Moreover, if the rate of suicide is considered a manifest indication of gender differences in the experience of distress, then as far as Britain is concerned, men now seem to be far more burdened by anxiety than women. The rate of suicide for men and women was roughly the same from 1911 to the early 1980s, however, since the 1980s the number of suicides among men has risen dramatically, while among women the number is falling. Men aged between 15 and 44 are now four times more likely than women to take their own lives (Kelly and Bunting 1998).

A number of studies have concluded that, traditionally, men have relied more than women on the institution of marriage for their relationships of emotional dependency (Belle 1991: 270). Except in the context of marriage, men appear to have fewer close confiding relationships than women (Thoits 1995a: 65), and thereby, it seems that they are more likely to be distressed by the growth in living alone. In Britain the proportion of men living alone who are under 30 is double that of women (Haskey 1996: 14) and John Charlton and colleagues hypothesise that at least half of the increase in male suicide may be explained with reference to the growing numbers of young men who either remain single or are going through a divorce (Charlton *et al.* 1993: 34; Kelly and Bunting 1998: 38). Moreover, they also consider the trends in suicide rates among young men to be related to the fact that this age-group stands at a higher risk of unemployment and is more prone to alcohol and drug abuse (Kelly *et al.* 1995).

Indeed, more recently researchers have begun to draw attention to the extent to which age appears to be a key variable within the social distribution of psychological distress (Turner and Marino 1994; Turner *et al.* 1995; Lazarus 1999: 165–89). While the most recent figures indicate a marginal decline in the numbers of male suicides, for British men below the age of 34 the rate continues to rise. Moreover, in marked contrast to older age groups, the rate of suicide among British women aged between 15 and 24 has also begun to rise (Kelly and Bunting 1998). R. Jay Turner and colleagues suggest that there is a growing consensus that young adults aged between 18 and 25 are most likely to develop a major neurotic disorder while the number of depressive symptoms decrease with age (Turner *et al.* 1995: 106–7 and 113–14). Similarly, Fred Cartmel and Andy Furlong refer to a range of studies which point to the conclusion that during the second half of the twentieth century the levels of psychological morbidity among young people in Great Britain have become 'substantially more prevalent' (Furlong and Cartmel 1997: 67–73). They suggest that this may not only be due to the increased uncertainty of the British labour market, but also a consequence of the increasing length of time it now takes for young people to make the transition between school and responsible adult life. Where more post-adolescents remain dependent upon their parents for housing and financial support, Cartmel and Furlong maintain that, especially where the structure of family life has become increasingly unstable (Haskey 1996; Simpson 1999), young adults are more likely to experience 'stressful conflicts and a lack of control over significant life events' (Furlong and Cartmel 1997).

The above evidence is taken by many to represent the 'core facts' as to the prevailing patterns of social distress. In the context of stress research, empirical sociologists have identified the objective social conditions and disruptive life-changing events which are most likely to be implicated in the development of mental health problems. On this basis, states of anxiety and depression, as expressed in symptoms of psychiatric morbidity, levels of alcohol dependency, drug abuse and the rate of suicide, are recognised as being unevenly distributed throughout the population. Moreover, there appears to be a clear association between the prevalence of psychological distress and the extent to which individuals are made vulnerable to the experience of unemployment, family conflict, the loss of intimacy and loneliness. Researchers largely agree that where studies use sample groups stratified by class, gender and age, then it is possible to identify clear patterns of social distress among men and women in similar socio-economic circumstances and at different stages in the life course. When it comes to describing the precise forms which these patterns take, then experts may reach marginally different conclusions depending upon the types of indicators which are used to measure the extent of psychiatric morbidity, nevertheless, majority opinion holds to the view that there are 'similar types and levels of stress among people who are exposed to similar social and economic conditions, who are incumbents in similar roles, and who come from similar situational contexts' (Pearlin 1989: 242).

In this context, it is recognised that there are well-established social indicators of anxiety. Where unemployment is high, job insecurity is rife, the divorce rate increases and people are unable to maintain close confiding relationships, then we should expect them to be particularly vulnerable to the experience of anxiety. Indeed, writers such as David Smail go so far as to identify the social experience of distress as the predictable result of government and managerial policies designed to subject work and family life to the rationalising force of the market economy (Smail 1999). For Smail, where the structural reorganisation of these social institutions takes place at a pace which denies people sufficient time and opportunity to secure their employment prospects, maintain their family relations and develop a new culture for negotiating with the revised meaning of their world, then we should expect to find large numbers of people in an acute state of personal distress.

However, as far as the prevalence of psychiatric morbidity is concerned, it is still only a minority of people in the most vulnerable groups who are prone to display symptoms which may be diagnosed as forms of mental illness. While there is a clear association between distressing life events and the onset of anxiety and depression, it seems clear that by focusing just upon the objective social conditions which shape the lives of those in vulnerable groups, we still do not possess a complete explanation for individuals' variable psychological responses to their location within the social system. Indeed, in official terms, the majority appear to remain in a relatively satisfactory state of 'health'. For example, in a series of studies which aim to demonstrate the aetiological significance of distressing life events within the onset of depression among British working-class women, George Brown and colleagues found that only 20 per cent of those who had recently experienced a crisis at work or in the home were liable to develop case level symptoms of psychiatric morbidity (Brown and Harris 1978; 1989; Brown *et al.* 1987; 1992). When seeking to identify the key variables which could account for the particular vulnerability of this group, they suggest that this ought to be considered not merely as a consequence of peculiarities in the objective social contexts in which people are made to live, but more specifically, as an affect of the meanings which they give to events in their lives. Accordingly, such studies have served to further alert researchers to the moderating force of meaning as the pivotal factor within the arousal of anxiety.

## The moderating force of meaning

Studies incorporating the *Social Readjustment Rating Scale* reveal that there is a broad consensus when it comes to identifying the most stressful types of life changing events (Miller and Rahe 1997). Following the pioneering work of Thomas Holmes and Richard Rahe (1967) researchers find that, when presented with a list of events which are widely recognised to involve people in the experience of distress, respondents are largely in agreement as to those which are most likely to have a disruptive impact upon our lives. However, it is important to recognise that the ways in which individuals evaluate the meanings of events in their own lives may not necessarily correspond with what they understand to be an accurate representation of events which are bad for society as a whole. Our shared understandings of the types of events which are most likely to arouse other people's anxiety, may well have little bearing upon the ways in which we negotiate the meanings of events in our own day-to-day experience of the world.

For example, following 'death of a spouse', most people rate 'divorce' as the most disruptive and potentially stressful event which may impact upon their lives (Holmes and Rahe 1967; Miller and Rahe 1997), however, where researchers such as Catherine Riessman have embarked upon qualitative studies of the personal meaning of divorce, they have found that this particular event may be interpreted as having a range of both positive and negative impacts upon people's lives (Riessman 1989;1990). Moreover, as to whether the personal experience of divorce has damaging effects upon our psychological health, it appears that a great deal depends upon the extent to which we interpret this event as 'undesirable' in relation to the ways in which we make sense of our past lives, current situation and future prospects. Indeed, it seems that it is the subjective meanings which are given to events which largely determine the extent to which people are liable to experience themselves as being in a state of distress. Accordingly, Leonard Pearlin advises:

> Not all circumstances, by any measure, can be judged as being stressors because of their inherent nature . . . The intensity and quality with which the same circumstances are experienced as stressors will vary with the meanings attached to the circumstances. For some, divorce is a fall from heaven, for others, a rescue from hell.
>
> (Pearlin 1991: 246–6)

When it comes to identifying those who are most likely to be anxious and distressed by divorce, it appears that it is not so much the objective fact of the event, but rather the subjective interpretation of its meaning which is vital for explaining how people actually *feel* in relation to their predicament. Thus, writers such as Robin Simon are inclined to suggest that where the majority of stress researchers have come to focus almost exclusively upon the objective social conditions which shape the lives of those in distress, a proper recognition of the moderating force of meaning upon people's vulnerability to anxiety and depression demands that they be more concerned to investigate the bearing of structural factors upon individual inclinations and opportunities to give positive meanings to events in their lives (Simon 1995; 1997).

Her own research focuses upon gender differences in the meanings given to role identities at work and in the home. In particular she is interested to highlight the extent to which men and women's differential vulnerability to distress may be significantly attributed to gender differences in the meanings which they give to the task of combining career commitments with parental duties. Married couples in similar jobs and with similar family commitments make sense of their roles in quite different ways. In particular, her in-depth interviews suggest that women are more likely than men to experience a conflict between the meaning of motherhood and the demands of the workplace. Simon claims that the social meaning of being a 'good' mother comes into conflict with the ways in which they experience their combined role of parent and employee to the extent to which they are more likely to feel guilty and depressed by the need to spend less time in the home for the sake of their work. Accordingly, she is inclined to explain gender differences in the experience of anxiety as a consequence of the contrasting ways in which men and women negotiate the meanings of their personal circumstances in relation to prevailing cultural values and beliefs about being a 'good' parent and spouse.

However, such conclusions rest upon a rather static conception of the meanings with which people make sense of their marital and occupational roles; there is no recognition of the potential for women to renegotiate the meanings of their lifestyle towards more positive conceptions of their combined parental and professional duties. While this study is concerned to highlight how the changing lifestyle of large numbers of white middle-class professionals may come into conflict with conventional values and beliefs about the 'good' mother and wife, it does not conceive of the extent to which this may also involve people in a cultural process where they are acquiring and creating new conventions for interpreting the meanings of their lives. Simon represents the cultures of parenthood and the workplace as fixed in time and space; she does not question their capacity for change.

Indeed, now that a great transformation is taking place in the structure of British family life we may have reached a point where, retrospectively, it becomes possible to trace the establishment of a new culture for making sense of our occupational and parental roles. With the falling rate of marriage, the growth in cohabitation, declining fertility, the rise in births outside marriage, and the majority of mothers now in paid employment, we are undoubtedly witnessing the development of a whole new set of 'family values' for the coming century (Haskey 1995; 1996; Shaw 1999; Shaw and Haskey 1999). Where the transition from the 'traditional' nuclear family to the 'unclear' family is understood by many to have involved people in a heightened experience of role insecurity (Simpson 1999), for others, this represents the positive development of a pioneering search for more fulfilling forms of intimacy and better ways of caring for our loved ones (Beck and Beck-Gernsheim 1995). Certainly, for many women, the decline of the 'traditional' nuclear family may be conceived as a sign of their liberation from gender roles in which they were denied a proper opportunity to express their individuality and were made to suffer the ideological force of patriarchal definitions of the 'good' housewife and mother.

The meaning of 'marriage' is open to a wide range of interpretations, and clearly, the perceived costs and benefits of entering into a married relationship appear to be considerably more varied in the 2000s than they were in the 1950s. The majority of young adults now *choose* to cohabit rather than marry, and further, while Great Britain has the highest divorce rate in Western Europe, the moral stigma of divorce seems more likely to be represented as an historical anachronism. Social attitudes towards intimacy appear to be in transition, and people are looking to alternative forms of relationships to meet their need for emotional support (Giddens 1992). While the basic fact remains that people's emotional well-being is heavily dependent upon their experience of social support (Thoits 1995a: 64–7), the types of relationships which are recognised as most conducive to intimacy may nowadays be more varied than in the middle decades of the last century. Indeed, Ray Pahl (1998) notes that there is evidence to suggest that people are increasingly inclined to rely upon friendships rather than family for the forms of psychological intimacy and social support which were the traditional preserve of marriage ties.

Such developments may well call for a substantial revision of some of the established conclusions of past research concerning the perceived benefits of marriage and negative impact of divorce and upon the prevalence of psychological distress (Gove and Hee-Choon 1989; Gove *et al.* 1990). Where the 'core facts' about the interrelationship between marriage, divorce, and psychological distress are revealed to be provisionally dependent upon the cultural forms through which we give meaning to our private lives, then we should anticipate the likelihood that these are liable to change with the times. The meanings of our personal relationships are embedded in cultural processes where, for the time being at least, it appears that increasing numbers of people are being made to renegotiate the terms of intimacy and re-evaluate the socio-emotional costs and benefits of 'traditional' types of family organisation.

Accordingly, where researchers have begun to focus upon the moderating force of meaning upon our vulnerability to psychological distress, this may not only serve to advance more detailed explanations of the interrelationship between structural conditions and their personal affects, but further, alert them to the extent to which the prevalence of anxiety is a cultural reality which is always open to change. As yet, few have ventured to conduct research into the social dynamics of the interrelationships between structural conditions, cultural formations and psychological states; the precise nature of the cultural mediation between social institutions and individual experiences of anxiety remains largely unexplored. However, where critical analysis is prepared to focus its attention upon the interaction between the cultural and the structural components of our distress, we may begin to piece together a greater understanding of the social constraints and opportunities which determine individuals' abilities to cope with their anxiety as a variable of meaning.

## Conclusion

In this chapter I have been inquiring into the possibility of measuring the level of anxiety among different sectors of the population, Moreover, I have been concerned to identify the types of social events and processes which, in the context of empirical research, appear to have a determining effect upon people's vulnerability to psychological distress. Insofar as I have been focusing upon the work of those concerned to account for the prevalence of anxiety as forms of psychiatric disorder, this most certainly should *not* be taken to represent an exhaustive account of its overall distribution throughout society. It is most likely that there are many alternative forms and expressions of anxiety, which while not officially interpreted as symptoms of 'disorder', are nevertheless, understood to comprise the general experience of malaise.

Throughout my discussion I have been particularly concerned to highlight the extent to which the possibility of identifying the presence of 'anxiety' in the words, bodily symptoms and behaviours of respondents requires researchers to commit themselves to a hermeneutical process in which one is liable to encounter a range of conflicting interpretations as to the proper meanings of the outward signs of our inner feelings. Moreover, where, for the sake of inter-study reliability, methodological frameworks are designed to discourage researchers from involving themselves in the idiosyncrasies of meaning which symptoms of distress hold for their respondents, this may force them into making interpretive commitments which fail to recognise the proper extent to which the problem of anxiety is encountered as a distressing affect of our subjective interpretations of our everyday experience of the world. Indeed, as stress researchers have identified the objective social conditions in which we are most likely to display symptoms of psychiatric morbidity, it appears that it is largely with reference to the forms of culture which give meanings to our personal circumstances that they are best able to explain individual variations in vulnerability to anxiety.

Where the experience of anxiety is understood to be moderated by the meanings which we give to events in our lives, I have argued that this may serve to alert researchers to the provisional character of any attempt at establishing the overall prevalence of this condition in society. Researchers may only provide us with snap-shot assessments of the interrelationship between structural conditions and their personal affects. Moreover, where all points of view are subject to a range of conflicting interpretations, they are also open to change. I am concerned to represent anxiety as a cultural reality which is embedded in social processes where there is always scope for individuals to acquire and create new meanings for the situations in which they find themselves. However, where I now turn to consider the task of coping, I would have us dwell in more detail upon the extent to which the ways in which the meaning of anxiety remains bound to the social circumstances in which we are made to live.

# 3

# Coping: from personal style to cultural critique

Anxiety functions to alert us to the fact that something is dangerously wrong with our world. The unpleasant quality of this experience agitates us into taking the necessary steps to remove ourselves from harm's way. Accordingly, one may identify anxiety as a necessary and normal part of the human condition. Anxiety has a purpose; it may serve above all else to protect those beliefs and practices which give meaning and value to our existence (May 1977). Moreover, on this view, it may well be conceived as the inspiration for artists and great thinkers to create new ways of giving form and expression to their life. Indeed, Kierkegaard contends that 'the more profoundly he is in anxiety, the greater is the man . . . [for] whoever is educated by anxiety is educated by possibility' (Kierkegaard 1980: 155–6).

However, for most of us, it seems the psychological trauma of this experience is more likely to be encountered as a frustrating burden rather than an opportunity to be educated in a higher meaning and purpose. We do not choose to court the 'adventure' of anxiety (ibid.), rather, so long as we are able, we are more likely to be committed to removing ourselves from any situation which causes us to feel this way. The abundance of popular literature devoted to the management of stress and anxiety testifies to the fact that large numbers of people find it extremely difficult to cope with their vulnerability to being in this condition. Generally speaking, anxiety is not welcomed as the inspiration for creative thinking, rather, it is encountered as a force in opposition to our well-being.

## ANXIETY IN A RISK SOCIETY

In this chapter I discuss some of the principal ways in which people may attempt to avoid or control anxiety so as to minimise its disruptive impact upon their lives. It is written in the conviction that it is only insofar as we are able to reach a critical vantage point from which to analyse our relative capacities for coping that we might begin to piece together a comprehensive framework to interpret the cultural meaning of anxiety. Moreover, I would further emphasise the extent to which the social distribution of anxiety is best explained in terms of the extent to which individuals have unequal access to the material, social and cultural resources which might empower them to allay their symptoms of distress.

Even where clinical psychology acknowledges the determining influence of a social environment upon our relative capacities for coping, the majority of writers remain committed to the view that if we are to feel more comfortable with our lives, then changes must take place in the ways in which we, as discrete individuals, think about and respond to the problems which cause us anxiety. In this context, our mental health is most likely to be represented as a strength of personality, rather than a matter of social endowment. The task of coping is held to begin with a change in our psychological orientation towards the world where the goal is to leave us better equipped to adapt to the prevailing status quo. Only a minority have ventured to question the logic of this premise so as to emphasise the extent to which the pathologies of our social environment are liable to deny us a form of culture which is sufficient to meet the demands of our day.

I shall be particularly concerned to present the task of coping as determined by social and cultural processes which are beyond the power of any single individual to control. On the one hand, this is to take the negative view that, left to our own resources we may never be in a position where we are able to completely rid ourselves of the feeling that something is deeply wrong with our lives, however, it is also to take the positive view that feeling anxious may be a right and proper response to the social reality in which we are made to live. Such an emphasis seeks to cast suspicion upon the notion that our anxieties stem from a weakness of individual personality, and rather, is designed to draw us towards a critical reflection upon the social origins of our mental and emotional well-being. Indeed, it may well be the case that by questioning society we do more to solve the problem of anxiety than can be achieved by persuading individuals that they might feel better if only they could come to a new way of 'seeing' their place in the world; for the language of personal pathology may actually serve to 'mystify' the proper meaning of our subjective experience of reality because it requires us to identify our thoughts and behaviours more as a product of individual character than an expression of the social and cultural conditions in which we find ourselves (Smail 1984; 1998;1999).

However, where the cultivation of a 'sociological imagination' may be identified as a necessary part of the process by which individuals come to a critical awareness of the extent to which the solution to the problem of anxiety lies in the direction of a change in the order of society, I would readily acknowledge that this may be judged to be woefully inadequate for enabling us to conceive the political means of changing the structural conditions which determine the course of our day-to-day lives. Indeed, reluctantly, I find myself convinced that as a matter of practical necessity we shall most likely be made to conceive the immediate task of coping in terms of the pervasive ideology of individualism. Nevertheless, following David Smail (1998), I would argue that where it is clear that our vulnerability to the experience of emotional distress is moderated by the forms of culture and society in which we are made to live, then it is primarily as a point of ethical responsibility that we can choose to make these the objects of our critical concern. Accordingly, where through the first two sections of this chapter I aim to highlight the extent to which our individual struggles to manage the burden of anxiety may be conceived as an expression of our location within the prevailing order of society, in the final section I offer a critical assessment of the value of sociology as an intellectual resource for the promotion of our psychological well-being.

## Seeking coherence and taking control

The literature on how we might best cope with our anxiety is vast, and any review is likely to be hindered by the fact that there is no consensus when it comes to using theoretical language to analyse the various modes of behaviour and cognition which are understood to help solve the problems which this condition inflicts upon our lives. Moreover, the range of terminology is confusing, and where often it appears that writers are using different words to mean the same thing, the same words also tend to appear in different theoretical contexts so that doubts may be raised as to whether they retain the same meaning. Nevertheless, at a broad level of comparison, most authorities are committed to the view that the task of coping begins in our minds.

When caught by anxiety we are left struggling to know how to think and what to do in order to keep ourselves from harm's way. We may perceive ourselves to be threatened by an unknown quantity of physical danger, however, it is often the case that the experience of anxiety is encountered in the context of a threat to our personal identity and self-esteem. On this view, our relative capacities for coping depend upon the extent to which we might possess a clearer understanding of what we need to do in order to protect ourselves from an anticipated danger, or rather, it is by acquiring a positive sense of purpose and belonging that we might moderate our feelings so as to keep anxiety at bay. If we are to better cope with anxiety then we must develop styles of thinking and behaviour which promote more consistency in attitudes and orientations, so that, when faced with the 'reality' of our situation, we might put our feelings in order and acquire the self-confidence to believe we have the power to solve our problems.

It is generally assumed that those who are best able to cope with their anxieties are liable to possess a 'sense of coherence' which promotes self-confidence and the belief that one is 'in control' of one's destiny (Antonovsky 1979). Indeed, more than any other factor, 'self-efficacy' or 'perceived control over life circumstances' has been identified as the most valuable coping resource and the foundation for our mental health (Aneshensel 1992; Thoits 1995a). John Mirowksy and Catherine Ross maintain that, 'of all the beliefs about self and society that might affect an individual's distress, belief in control over one's life may be the most important' (Mirowsky and Ross 1986: 26). It is presumed that high self-esteem and a sense of mastery not only serve 'to buffer the negative health effects of stress' (Thoits 1995a: 60), but also increase the likelihood that an individual will be empowered to adopt problem-solving strategies for removing themselves from the situations which cause them to enter into the condition of anxiety (Aneshensel 1992: 28).

Accordingly, in the majority of cases, the ideal solution to the problem of anxiety is conceived in terms of the extent to which we might possess a style of reasoning which has the power to free us from our agitated state of uncertainty; the more we are convinced of our power to control the course of our lives, the less likely it is that we shall be overwhelmed by feelings of anxiety. However, it is a largely incontrovertible fact that large numbers of people find it extremely difficult to think and feel this way. Many (most?) of us are all too frequently made to be aware of the extent to which we are lacking self-confidence and feel limited in our capacity to control the situations which cause us to experience anxiety. Indeed, I suspect that there are occasions where we would all gladly embrace the opportunity to feel a bit more self-assured.

Self-efficacy appears to be a limited resource and an extensive literature on coping has developed with the aim of identifying the particular attributes which enable an individual to conceive the experience of anxiety more as a challenge to find creative solutions to their problems than as a sign of powerlessness and defeat (Lazarus and Folkman 1984; Monat and Lazarus 1991). Insofar as the majority of research is informed by the traditions of psychoanalytic ego psychology, an emphasis tends to be placed upon the extent to which coping is a product of our *individual* modes of cognition and emotional processing abilities (Lazarus and Folkman 1984: 117–40). Considerable efforts have been made to detail the dimensions of the cognitive processes which enable some people to be particularly skilled at managing their symptoms of distress (Cohen 1991). In this context, effective coping is far more likely to be identified as a disposition or trait of personality than a matter of socio-economic and cultural endowment (Vaillant 1977).

For example, where Richard Lazarus is prepared to recognise that our personal resources for coping may be influenced by our cultural beliefs about the nature of self and society, he is inclined to place greater emphasis upon the extent to which some people are simply born better equipped than others with the psychological attributes to 'adapt' to stressful stimuli. In addition to this, he suggests that it may be during the early years of childhood that we are liable to develop a personal style of coping which is largely unamenable to change in later life (Lazarus 1999: 61–72). Likewise, Salvatore Maddi and Suzanne Kobasa argue that parent–child interactions are what matter most for the development of 'hardiness' towards stress. Moreover, they are inclined to consider a person's socio-economic background as largely irrelevant for whether they have developed a mental aptitude for coping with the experience of anxiety. On this view, our financial position or social standing is understood to have no bearing upon the extent to which we might provide our children with a family 'atmosphere' which enables them to feel in control of their lives and acquire the self-confidence to set about solving their personal problems. As far as these writers are concerned, so long as we are lucky enough to have parents who are disposed to provide us with love and support, then we may acquire the positive traits of personality which are best suited to equip us with a sense of mastery when faced with the problems of our social environment (Maddi and Kobasa 1991).

As a matter of temperament or childhood conditioning, certain 'types' of people are hereby considered to be disposed to experience more anxiety than others. Moreover, where some individuals are prone to develop forms of neurosis which are categorised as a 'disorder' of personality, there is no agreement as to how far they may be able to modify their cognitive styles and behaviour so as to make them more adaptable to the stress of life. Nevertheless, most experts in the field of mental health hold to the view that it may at least be possible to teach them some styles of thinking and behaviour which will enable them to exercise more control over their symptoms of distress. Susan Folkman and colleagues suggest that there are two main ways in which experts might 'intervene' in the lives of people in distress so as to help them improve their capacity for coping (Folkman *et al.* 1991). In the first place, an attempt may be made to empower an individual to act upon their social environment so as to remove the particular problems which cause them anxiety. However, insofar as it is often the case that individuals can do little to change or control their personal circumstances, then efforts may be focused upon helping them to better manage their emotional response towards the 'reality' in which they find themselves. As far as the latter is concerned, it is generally understood that so long as it is possible to make the world *appear* less hostile and intimidating, then we may at least be able to enhance our capacity to keep the worst effects of anxiety under control.

In this context a 'problem-focused' intervention may involve teaching a person to organise their time and social commitments more effectively so as to enable them to minimise the stress of work. In addition to this, they may be trained to be more assertive or taught a decision-making strategy whereby it becomes possible for them to identify their personal goals and take the necessary steps to realise their ambitions. Alternatively, it could involve them seeking social support or taking advice so as to resolve a problem of interpersonal conflict. Moreover, insofar as their symptoms of anxiety may be exacerbated by a poor state of physical health, they may be advised to exercise more, stop smoking, cut down their alcohol consumption, eat a healthy diet and get more sleep (Powell and Enright 1990).

While various relaxation techniques or psychotropic drugs may be prescribed as a means of controlling the most severe symptoms of distress, the majority of 'emotion-focused' interventions are inclined to use some kind of cognitive therapy as a means of helping people to moderate the affects of their negative emotions. For example, insofar as the experience of anxiety may be aroused as a consequence of negative self-defeating thought processes, Donald Meichenbaum's 'self-intructional' techniques aim to teach people to think more positively about their lives so as to 'inoculate' themselves against the experience of stress (Meichenbaum 1977; Meichenbaum and Cameron 1983). Moreover, it is by challenging a person's 'illogical' interpretations of the situations which cause them distress that therapists such as Aaron Beck aim to 'restructure' their clients' processes of cognition towards a more positive appraisal of their capacity to control their symptoms of distress (Beck 1976; Beck *et al.* 1985). Such methods work according to the assumption that the most severe symptoms of neurotic disorder are largely the result of a faulty process of reasoning which leads an individual to overestimate the reality of a prospective danger and underestimate their capacity to keep themselves from harm's way. Having identified the cognitive 'errors' which cause them to misapprehend the 'reality' of their circumstances, the aim is to introduce them to alternative frameworks of understanding which can be used to construct a new relational meaning towards the problems which place them in distress. On this view, it is hoped that where an individual might be equipped with an appraisal of reality which corrects their 'distorted' view of the world, then they might begin to behave with more self-confidence so as to feel less anxious and distressed.

The coping literature is overwhelmingly committed to helping individuals to live with the stresses of their social environment according to the limitations of their adaptational resources. Accordingly, where most of us are understood to be born with a form of mentality which may be nurtured to equip us with styles of coping which permit us to lead a relatively 'normal' life, an unfortunate minority are identified as having inherited or acquired a form of temperament which disposes them to feel less confident to solve their problems and to possess a greater inclination to perceive themselves as a person 'in danger'. On this view, one might well be inclined to suggest that the 'types' of people who possess the strength of character for dealing with stress are most likely to make a success of their education and take control of their lives so as to occupy positions of power and material prosperity, while those individuals who are less able to adapt to the pressures of life will find themselves in low-status jobs where their daily routine is more likely to be governed by circumstances beyond their control. Indeed, where stress researchers have turned to inquire into social patterns of coping behaviour they have found evidence which may be interpreted to support such a proposition.

## Social patterns of coping

There is now a considerable amount of accumulated evidence to suggest that men and women in similar socio-economic circumstances who perform similar social roles are liable to display largely the same types of coping behaviours and problem-solving strategies. In the context of sociological stress research, it is widely accepted that 'mastery varies inversely with socioeconomic status' (Aneshensel 1992: 27). The lower classes consistently report more feelings of powerlessness and appear to be more pessimistic about their ability to change their lives for the better (Mirowsky and Ross 1989; Turner and Roszell 1994). Moreover, it is well established that men are more likely than women to report feeling high self-esteem and are more frequently observed to deal with stress by adopting rational problem-solving strategies which draw upon their independent powers of self-control. By contrast, where women are observed to respond to the experience of anxiety by discussing their problems with others so as to better manage their emotions, they are understood to be less inclined to make individual efforts to exercise control over the stressful events in their lives (Belle 1991; Thoits 1991).

Accordingly, one might well suppose that the types of people who are least 'adaptable' to living in the modern world are most likely to find themselves among the lower classes, and men are more 'naturally' inclined than women to develop a psychological orientation towards the world which disposes them to adopt rational problem-solving strategies as a means of dealing with their symptoms of distress. Indeed, where the coping literature seeks to emphasise the extent to which a sense of mastery and self-control are acquired as a 'trait' of personality, it seems logical to interpret social patterns of coping not so much as evidence for the determining influence of society upon the individual, but rather, as a result of the ways in which individuals are disposed to make their society. However, few would go so far as to dismiss the possibility of understanding our relative capacities for coping as an expression of the socio-economic and cultural conditions in which we are made to live.

Indeed, some commentators would rather place an emphasis upon the extent to which individuals in low-paid low-status jobs are not only denied the financial resources to effect positive changes to their lifestyle, but also, in a culture which places a high value on material success, are likely to suffer low self-esteem and be more inclined towards fatalism (Mirowsky and Ross 1986: 30; Locke and Taylor 1991; Wilkinson 1996; 1999). Given the cultural significance of paid employment for role identity and a sense of personal achievement, it is understood that so long as these groups suffer more job insecurity and higher rates of unemployment, then they will most likely be *made* to lack self-confidence and struggle to maintain a positive meaning for their lives (Fryer 1995). Moreover, where lower income groups and the unemployed are more likely to smoke heavily and drink excessive amounts of alcohol (Acheson 1998: 16), this may be understood not so much as a consequence of the extent to which they are individually disposed to develop an addiction to drugs, but rather, as an indication of the extent to which the poverty of their material and cultural circumstances denies them the opportunity of adopting a more 'healthy' problem-solving style of coping with their immediate problems of day-to-day life

(Graham 1987; Wilkinson 1996: 185–90; Jarvis and Wardle 1999). Indeed, David Fryer contends that where longitudinal studies such as that conducted by Dooley and colleagues (1992) find that people usually begin drinking excessively in response to problems at work, we should consider the experience of unemployment and job insecurity to be not so much a result, but rather the *cause* of their psychological vulnerability to distress (Fryer 1995: 266).

Likewise, it is possible to explain the contrasting ways in which men and women tend to respond to the experience of distress more as a product of socio-economic and cultural determination than as a reflection of innate differences between the sexes. In the first place, where most women have more intimate relationships than men and are more inclined to seek emotional support from others as a means of coping with their anxieties, this may be understood as the inevitable consequence of the extent to which they are subjected to a process of socialisation where at every stage of the life cycle they are more likely to be cast in the role of 'comforter', 'counsellor' and 'companion' (Gore and Colten 1991: 150). In Western culture help-seeking and the disclosure of feelings are stereo-typically portrayed as female behaviours, and as such, are more likely to be adopted by women (Belle 1991).

However, one might also explain women's emotion-focused coping style as the result of the extent to which their position in the labour market and their social role in the home are liable to *make* them more vulnerable to the distress of social and economic deprivation. There are twice as many women as men in temporary forms of employment (with low pay and poor working conditions) and they are five times more likely than men to be in part-time work. Taking all sources of independent income into account, women have only half as much money as men (CSO 1995). Moreover, insofar as occupying the role of 'mother' or 'housewife' leaves many women economically dependent on men, then it is suggested that they are more likely to feel a sense of powerlessness and low self-esteem (Mirowsky and Ross 1986: 27–8). Accordingly, women's help-seeking behaviour may be understood as a consequence of the fact that they are less likely than men to possess the material and social resources which would afford them the possibility of acting independently so as to achieve positive solutions to their problems; where they are unable to assume control over the situations which cause them distress, women cope by sharing their problems so that by venting their feelings they might at least experience a level of emotional catharsis (Thoits 1991).

Similarly, one might understand the 'typically' male style of coping, not only as the result of the extent to which they are culturally disposed to portray themselves as self-assured, independent and in control of their emotions, but

73

also as a consequence of the fact that they are likely to perform social roles where there are more opportunities to use rational problem-solving as a means of alleviating their symptoms of distress. For instance, Deborah Belle notes that men tend to regard help-seeking as a sign of weakness which is liable to be penalised in a world of work where 'success' depends upon maintaining a façade of self-confidence and cool control (Belle 1991: 264–5). However, insofar as they are also more likely to occupy positions of power in the workplace and possess the material resources with which to act to change their environment, then their stoical independent style of coping may be understood to be determined more by a collective experience of social privilege than innate psychology.

Indeed, where women come to experience more financially rewarding forms of employment, they have been shown to acquire more feelings of self-confidence and exhibit a greater sense of being in control of their personal circumstances (Downey and Moen 1987). Furthermore, Peggy Thoits found that where her research used a sample of middle-class college students, then both men and women tended to exhibit a similarly high level of self-efficacy (Thoits 1991). By contrast, where men are consistently made to experience the afflictions of economic and social deprivation, then they are also observed to develop a more expressive style of coping which relies more heavily upon the emotional support of social networks (Ulbrich et al. 1989). Indeed, gender appears to have little bearing upon the extent to which the experience of poverty and downward social mobility is liable to erode a person's self-esteem and leave them feeling powerless to bring about a positive change in their life circumstances (Fryer 1995).

In recent years, Richard Wilkinson has gone further than most to identify our vulnerability to anxiety as being largely conditioned by the experience of relative deprivation. By comparing the rates of stress-related mortality in Sweden, Japan, Britain and the United States, he notes that there is now a substantial amount of empirical research to indicate a clear association between levels of income inequality and the overall prevalence of 'psychosocial' distress (Wilkinson 1996: 72–109). Where Japan and Sweden have higher rates of life expectancy and lowest rates of infant mortality, he maintains that this is substantially due to the extent to which these societies have been shaped by an ethos of egalitarianism which makes people more resilient towards the experience of depression and anxiety. Conversely, he explains the widening health gap in Britain and the United States as a consequence of increasing income inequalities which leave large numbers of people feeling ever more desperate, bitter and devalued. Where the damaged health of lower income groups may be exacerbated by factors such as a poor diet and bad housing, Wilkinson would rather place an emphasis upon the extent to which this is a result of the social, psychological and emotional deprivation that is experienced in relation to the negative meanings which these people acquire and create for their lives (Wilkinson 1999).

On this view a chronic experience of anxiety, insecurity and helplessness is identified as a cultural product of life in low-income households. Equally the possibility of conceiving oneself as a person with social value who is in control of their lives is considered to be culturally determined by a position of privilege within the social hierarchy. Moreover, insofar as income equality appears to be a major contributing factor to the overall level of social integration and moral solidarity in a society, then there are further benefits to be gained for making us more resilient towards anxiety. It is not only the case that where people perceive themselves to be surrounded by supportive relationships, they are liable to feel better equipped to cope with symptoms of distress (Eckenrode 1991: 4–6; Thoits 1995a: 64–7), but also a strong sense of social solidarity appears to con-tribute to a lowering of the crime rate, fewer numbers of road accidents, and a lower rate of divorce (Wilkinson 1996: 153–72). Indeed, it may well be the case that where governments act to improve the levels of income equality in their societies, they will not only be placing greater numbers of people in a position to acquire the cultural resources for coping with the experience of distress, but they also will reduce the incidence of some of the problematic events which are known to arouse our anxiety.

Accordingly, where there is now a developed tradition of empirical research which reveals an unequal distribution of coping resources within and between developed societies, there is no shortage of commentators who are prepared to argue that this is most clearly explained as evidence of conceiving our resilience towards anxiety more as an expression of social endowment rather than as a matter of personal disposition. This is not to deny that some part of the problem of anxiety may be attributed to factors of personality, but it is to place the greater emphasis upon the extent to which an individual is liable to experience and respond to their anxiety according to the social conditions in which they are made to live. Moreover, it leads to the strong suggestion that where the literature on coping tends to concentrate overwhelmingly upon the extent to which it may be possible for individuals to better adapt to the stress of life in modern societies, then this leaves the major part of the problem of anxiety outside their field of analysis. Where experts look for change at the level of individual personality, they should rather be looking for a change in society.

## The sane society

In the middle decades of the last century Erich Fromm may well be identified as having worked most consistently to bring psychologists towards a fuller recognition of the extent to which the experience of anxiety results not so much from weaknesses in our innate capacities for coping, but more as a response to the socio-economic and cultural conditions in which we find ourselves. For the purposes of critical analysis, he proposes that it is possible for us to identify our thoughts, feelings and actions as being determined by 'ideal-types' of *social character* which develop as a product of our shared experiences of day-to-day life (Fromm 1942: 239–53; 1947: 54–117; Fromm and Maccoby 1970). A social character functions to provide us with a common way of relating towards the world; that is, it conditions us into 'seeing' certain attitudes and forms of behaviour as both rational and desirable. Moreover, Fromm would further emphasise that it is through a dominant form of social character that a society moulds individuals into 'wanting to act as they have to act' so as to preserve the prevailing economic order and the way of life it sustains (Fromm 1956: 79). Accordingly, where it is possible to identify groups of people who are committed to a shared understanding of the truth, meaning and morality of their relationships at work and in the home, he would direct us towards the extent to which this conforms to the dominant socio-economic and political interests of society.

Fromm presents us with a conception of human history which identifies the dynamics of social character as the key to explaining the different ways in which people make their culture and develop a specific psychological and ethical orientation towards the world. However, while emphasising the extent to which character is made to adapt to society by the lure of ideology combined with the brute force of economic power, he also maintains that we possess some basic existential needs which, when left unsatisfied, may cause us to 'react' against the social conditions in which we find ourselves so as to make them more adaptable to our 'human nature'. He argues that:

> in speaking of the socio-economic structure of society moulding man's character, we speak only of one pole in the interconnection between social organization and man. The other pole to be considered is man's nature, moulding in turn the social conditions in which he lives . . . While it is true that man can adapt himself to almost any conditions, he is not a blank sheet of paper on which culture writes its text. Needs like the striving for happiness, harmony, love and freedom

are inherent in his nature. They are also dynamic factors in the historical process which, if frustrated, tend to arouse psychic reactions,
ultimately creating the very conditions suited to original strivings.

(Fromm 1956: 81)

Accordingly, his critical analysis of the condition of anxiety in the context of
industrial capitalism is designed to advance a dialectical theory of the relationship between 'man' and society. Where on the one hand, he considers humanity
to be striving to attain a level of 'mental health' which expresses itself in loving
relationships, creative work, a clear sense of identity, democratic systems of
government and a form of morality which seeks to place the good of the collective above that of the (egoistic) individual, on the other hand, he presents
society as always working to subordinate our lives to forms of economy and culture which are liable to leave us fearful and resentful of each other and with a
disposition to feel helpless and unfulfilled. Moreover, as the antagonism
between the psychological needs of our 'nature' and the demands of society
gives rise to an historical process in which each stage of our social development
may be conceived as a temporary solution to the problem of subordinating the
former to the latter, he believes that it becomes possible to discern some clues
as to the type of social conditions in which we are most likely to acquire forms
of character for feeling 'at home' in the world.

In *The Sane Society* (1956) he is totally uncompromising when arguing that
a potential cure for our 'social pathology' can only be brought into effect when
a simultaneous change takes place in every sphere of our social, political, economic and cultural activity, for he is adamant that 'the concentration of effort in
any of these spheres, to the exclusion or neglect of others, is destructive of all
changes' (ibid.: 271). Accordingly, where he identifies the principle of 'com-
munitarian socialism' as a guideline for detailing a way of life through which
we might attain full mental health, he seeks nothing else besides a wholesale
transformation of every dimension of society. To this end, Fromm conceives the
route towards our sanity to require workers to be empowered to participate in
the management of industry, an extensive system of adult education, a fully
democratised political system, the abolition of world poverty, equality of
income, collective forms of art and a universal 'religion' based upon the ethical
principles of humanism (ibid.: 321–52). On this view, the course of history
points towards the real possibility of achieving an alternative form of society
beyond Western capitalism and Soviet-style communism in which the 'alienated' condition of our humanity is abolished in an entirely new way of life.
Moreover, he presents this not only as a matter of political choice, but further,

as the necessary course of action for bringing our history of 'dehumanisation' to a new human beginning.

Where Fromm ventures to prescribe a cure for our 'social pathology' he considers nothing else besides the perfect society as offering us the possibility of experiencing full mental health. Accordingly, when it comes to considering the extent to which our powers of coping are limited by the social conditions in which we find ourselves, he must surely be identified as advocating not only the most uncompromising, but also, the most highly idealistic solution to the problem of living with anxiety. As such, his theories have always been criticised for their utopianism (Briggs 1956; Hausdorff 1972: 88–94). Moreover, where now Fromm's contribution to our understanding of life in capitalist society is seldom recognised in the context of academic scholarship, then this may be explained not only in terms of the extent to which it has become intellectually unfashionable to express faith in the progressive potential of 'human nature' (Rickert 1986: 388), but further, as a consequence of the widespread conviction that socialism may no longer be considered a viable alternative to capitalism (Kumar 1993; 1995).

In the wake of the collapse of communism it is now unusual to find social commentators who are prepared to countenance the notion that Western modernity might be directed towards a stage of development beyond that of global capitalism. For the foreseeable future, the majority of sociologists appear to be resigned to living in a society which is dominated by the drive to sustain economic growth and where most people are unquestioning in their commitment towards consumerism. Where great changes appear to be taking place in the organisation of work and family life, in the final analysis, most would identify these as reactions to discontinuities in the organisation of capitalist economies which are strengthening the power of the global marketplace to dictate the course of our lives. Indeed, while we might live to witness the development of new and possibly more ruthless forms of capitalism, most analysts hold to the view that we have entered a period of human history in which it has become inconceivable for national governments to choose an alternative course of modernisation, and all the more so if this is held to involve a return to the principles of traditional forms of socialism (Lash and Urry 1987; 1994; Fukuyama 1989; Hall and Jacques 1989; Bauman 1992: 175–86; 1999; Giddens 1994b; Hutton and Giddens 2000).

From the critical perspective of writers such as Fromm, this is to resign ourselves to a lifestyle structured by forms of economy, culture and society which will always leave us prone to anxiety and do damage to our personal relationships. On this point there is widespread agreement among the sociological community. So long as the development of 'civilisation' is bound to the dynamics of global capitalism, there appears to be little doubting the fact that more profound social inequalities, inevitable economic instability, and a burgeoning ecological crisis are liable to leave large numbers of people anxiously distressed by the condition of their lives. Indeed, perhaps it is now more than ever that we are in a position to recognise that where industrial capitalism thrives upon 'a constantly expanding market', 'the constant revolutionizing of production' and the 'uninterrupted disturbance of all social conditions', then a future of 'everlasting uncertainty and agitation' is guaranteed (Marx 1977: 224). The point at which contemporary analysis begins to depart from the traditions of critical theory is with regard to the very possibility of a population facing up to their way of life with 'sober senses' so that alternative forms of social organisation are identified as a real political choice.

If this is a correct interpretation of our state of 'civilisation' at this point in history, what is left for sociology to offer in terms of a solution to the problem of anxiety? Indeed, is it even right to represent sociology as a discipline which should aspire to legislate on behalf of the order of society (Bauman 1987)? Should we simply be content to consider the tools of sociological inquiry as a hermeneutical resource for the seemingly ever more complex task of describing 'the way things are'? Accordingly, while 'the sociological imagination' might still be celebrated as a means of relating public issues of structure to the personal problems of day-to-day life, should it give up on its 'promise' to inspire us to find ways of changing our lives for the better (Mills 1959)?

Certainly, in the context of stress research it appears that sociology has little purpose beyond providing commentators with a set of concepts for describing the structured patterns of distress in modern societies (Mirowsky and Ross 1986; Pearlin 1989; Eckenrode 1991; Aneshensel et al. 1991; Aneshensel 1992; Turner et al. 1995; Thoits 1995a: 56). Where it may be used to reveal the types of social conditions in which people are most likely to display symptoms of distress, in the vast majority of cases there is no attempt to relate such information to a critical theory of modernity which places the order of society in question. For example, having provided her readers with a summary review of the research which details the social distribution of stress in modern societies, Carol Aneshensel does no more than conclude that:

> The occurrence of systematic stress is not necessarily an indication of a social system run amok but may reflect instead the system functioning precisely as it is supposed to function. For example, a capitalist free-enterprise system inevitably produces business failure;

the sole questions are which industries falter and what occupations encounter contracting employment opportunities. The imperatives associated with maintenance of the social system inevitably create tension between the individual and the collectivity . . . Systematic conditions of tension are more prevalent among some social groups than others, largely as a consequence of inequality in the distributive system.

(Aneshensel 1992: 33)

Moreover, where stress researchers may go so far as to conceive the experience of distress as the predictable response to the structural conditions which determine our 'choice' of lifestyle, when it comes to the task of coping, their critical focus is directed almost exclusively upon the psychosocial attributes of 'the individual' rather than the forms of social organisation in which they are made to live. Indeed, even where writers such as Leonard Pearlin would alert his colleagues to the extent to which 'research provides little justification for an unbridled enthusiasm for the power of coping in the stress process' (Pearlin 1991: 274), practitioners appear to remain convinced that when attempts are made to 'intervene' in this process, they should be committed to helping individuals to better adapt to the prevailing order of society (Folkman *et al.* 1991). Accordingly, where the problem of distress might be recognised as having a social aetiology, it seems that most remain committed to the view that resources for coping are acquired as a strength of personality.

However, for David Smail, this is to deny sociology an ethical role which is indispensable in helping people to confront the brute facts about their experiences of distress. He rejects any attempt to represent the task of coping in terms of helping the individual to better adjust themselves to the status quo insofar as this encourages us to interpret anxiety more as an indication of personal weakness than as the proper response to the social conditions in which we are made to live (Smail 1984). Smail argues that so long as the order of society is conceived as some kind of 'impersonal necessity' which is beyond our power to change, then this is not only to 'mystify' the extent to which the world is organised as matter of political decision, but further, it is to leave unquestioned an ideology of individualism which, while persuading us to believe that there is nothing we can do about the state of society, leaves us convinced that it is *only* by individual strength of will that we might better cope with our personal problems (Smail 1998; 1999). Accordingly, he suggests that critical sociology should be identified as a therapeutic resource to enable people to break free from the deceptive mythology that they are in need of some kind of 'treatment' so that they might acknowledge the significance of anxiety as a sign that we must call society into question.

It may now be impossible to conceive, let alone create social conditions in which there is no exploitation, greed and abuse of power, nevertheless, the weight of sociological research points towards the conclusion that until society is transformed in this direction then we shall always be vulnerable to the experience of emotional distress and anxiety. While Smail seeks to distance himself from any optimistic prognosis for our future, he considers it vitally important that we face up to the sociologically revealed reality of our situation so as to confront the social pathologies of our times. Indeed, he is adamant that if we are to make any progress towards a solution to the problem of anxiety then every effort must be made to create a public space in which it becomes possible to inquire into the *morality* of the forms of social organisation which cause us to feel this way. Accordingly, he celebrates social critics such as Pierre Bourdieu (1984) and Jürgen Habermas (1990) for the extent to which their work contributes to a history of ethical discourse which seeks 'to combat and contain forms of conduct envisaged as ineradicable' (Smail 1998: 151; 1999). Smail maintains that:

> if one is to be able to understand the processes whereby people become unable to realise their potentialities in public living, to learn how to make a bodily contribution to the social world, to treat each other with kindness and forbearance as ends rather than means, and to become, as it were, the organic custodians of an unknowable future, the ability ethically to criticize the social structures in which we live is one which will have actively to be preserved. Not, of course, that the ability to make moral judgements will of itself change the world, but it is certainly the prerequisite to the kind of moral and political action by which the actual structures and institutions may be altered . . . an impotent recognition of moral failure is in my view preferable to a misguided trust in technical solutions which serve to justify further abuses.
>
> (Smail 1998: 152)

A similar argument is to be found in Zygmunt Bauman's attempt to outline a solution to the problem of poverty in a consumer society (Bauman 1998). While characteristically pessimistic with regard to the future possibility that humanity might work to create a social order which does more than treat its poor as 'problem people' with no value as potential consumers, Bauman maintains that now more than ever we need to work at preserving the critical tradition of putting society in question. Accordingly, while he recognises that it is all too easy to judge Claus Offe as being 'irrealistic' for proposing that social justice requires us to 'decouple' income entitlement from individual earning capacity (Offe 1996: 210), nevertheless, he considers it a matter of ethical responsibility for sociologists to alert society to the fact that if we are to commit ourselves to the construction of more humane forms of social organisation, we must first be prepared to imagine the possibility of living in a radically different world.

Indeed, it is for this reason that Richard Wilkinson argues that if we are to work at reducing the negative health effects of income distribution, then egalitarianism must be instituted as our prime societal goal (Wilkinson 1996; 1999). He maintains that where it is becoming increasingly clear that there is a direct link between relative poverty and the social distribution of emotional distress, then the 'first step' towards finding a solution to the problem of anxiety must be for politicians to recognise that wherever the pursuit of economic growth leads to a breakdown in social cohesion and greater inequalities in wealth and privilege, then this is bound to have a corrosive effect upon the mental and physical health of the nation. Moreover, while he believes that it is now highly improbable that societies might be convinced to break faith with the notion that our fulfilment is to be found in ever-increasing levels of material consumption, once again, it is out of an ethical commitment to the value of 'human dignity' that Wilkinson proposes that, if we are to be optimistic for the future of our 'civilisation', then 'economic management must have the explicit aim of increasing social cohesion and the social quality of life' (Wilkinson 1996: 223).

Accordingly, while traditional approaches to understanding the historical processes which gave rise to modern societies may now be judged to be inadequate for grappling with the 'new uncertainties' and complexities of social life in an age of globalisation (Hutton and Giddens 2000), ultimately, it is as a matter of moral concern that some would uphold the imaginative struggle to apply reason to the task of achieving a way of life which does full justice to the value of our humanity. Indeed, where the ethical imperative which inspires the work of criticism is openly acknowledged by Erich Fromm, then on this point at least, there is a strong line of continuity between his quest for the 'sane society' and the more 'intellectually embarrassed' forms of critical resistance which appear in the works of writers such as Bauman and Smail. Nevertheless, there can be little doubting the fact that at the turn of the new century, the possibility of achieving a solution to the problem of anxiety in a change of society is unlikely to be judged as anything else but extremely remote. Therefore, it seems that, for now at least, there may be no choice but to confront the *immediate* task of coping as a problem of our individuality. Indeed, when confronted with the daily challenge of managing symptoms of distress, even those who object to such an approach at the point of intellectual debate, will most likely find themselves practically subscribing to an ideology of individualism. However, writing as a sociologist with an ethical commitment to the work of criticism, I find myself agreeing wholeheartedly with David Smail when he advises that, 'even though we may be sure that [this] will involve us in the greatest difficulty, we cannot possibly foretell what our endeavours may lead to' (Smail 1998: 159–60).

## Conclusion

To note the moral virtue of social criticism as a resource for coping may be considered as no more than a piecemeal contribution to the task of finding a solution to the problem of anxiety. Indeed, it may even be dismissed as ill-considered and naïve. For where we may be identified as living in an age where there is a crisis of moral certainty (Macintyre 1985; 1988), such proposals will always be vulnerable to the criticism that so long as we are unable to agree upon the rational criteria for pronouncing ethical judgements upon the order of society, then the question of 'whose justice [and] which rationality?' will remain to pour scorn upon the aspirations of sociological radicalism (Crook 1991). Accordingly, where we look towards morality as the justification for calling society into question, we may be judged to do no more than subject ourselves to a range of intellectually agonising questions which will probably do more to arouse than allay our anxieties. However, insofar as our capacity for moral responsibility may be identified as the greatest reason for hoping we can make real a form of society in which anxiety does no more than lead us to realise the full potential of all that is best in our humanity (Bauman 1993), then surely (albeit in 'fear and trembling'), the questioning must continue?

Indeed, the moral impulse to question the relationship between society and anxiety should be recognised as a major factor contributing to the development of 'the risk debate' in the social sciences. Where over the last three chapters I have been concerned to develop a sociological conception of the experience of anxiety in contemporary societies, then this has been with the purpose of providing the reader with a set of critical questions for exploring the contrasting ways in which the concept of risk might now be used to account for the problems which this condition inflicts upon our lives. Accordingly, in what follows

I will argue that the task of coping with anxiety, is just *one* dimension to the process of experiencing distress which can be used to develop an interpretation of the cultural significance of 'risk consciousness' in our times. Moreover, where elsewhere I have explored the problem of establishing a definitive meaning for anxiety, as well as the extent to which it may be conceived as a product of the social and cultural conditions in which we are made to live, then this is with the aim of identifying contrasting roles for the concept of risk within sociological narratives on the origins of our current 'age of anxiety'. Insofar as an ongoing controversy surrounds the possibility of establishing a clear understanding of the constituent aspects and possible causes of anxiety, as well as the best methods of coping with this condition, then I would argue that this might be used as a critical vantage point for explaining conflicting interpretations of the prominence of 'risk' in the public sphere and as a matter of academic debate. Indeed, I am inclined to suggest that where we come to recognise that there can be no final certainty with regard to the meaning of the relationship between anxiety and 'risk consciousness', then we are in a better position to explain the cultural and political significance of these particular ways of feeling and thinking about our world.

Part II

# Anxiety and risk

# 4

## Anxiety in relation to risk

Where people are made vulnerable to the 'problem of anxiety' they are liable to encounter difficult questions concerning how they should make sense of this experience and how they might act so as to alleviate their symptoms of distress. So long as we remain 'in anxiety', then I understand this as a sign that we have yet to acquire the knowledge which is sufficient to allow us to define the full dimensions of the causes of our emotional distress, and thereby we are left struggling to identify a clear course of action which might lead us to feel more secure and 'at home' in the world. Indeed, following Freud (1979: 324–9) I have presented the trauma of anxiety as functioning for the purpose of 'seeing' our way through a situation of foreboding obscurity so that, by illuminating the 'reality' of an anticipated danger, we might take the necessary steps to remove ourselves from harm's way. In the context of the analytical distinction between fear and anxiety (see Chapter 1), where fears are understood to always 'refer to something definite' (Kierkegaard 1980: 42) and anxiety is held to have 'a quality of indefiniteness and a lack of object' (Freud 1979: 325), one might conceive this experience of trauma to have the aim of transforming the agitated uncertainty of anxiety into the sure knowledge of fear.

By placing a particular emphasis upon the extent to which the experience of anxiety can be identified as thriving upon the tension between our knowledge and ignorance of fearful situations, I am concerned to draw the reader's attention to the possibility of understanding this particular mode of being as not only conditioned by the cultural context in which we find ourselves, but also as a problem of culture. Where anxiety prevails, there is always a struggle for coherence and purpose. Indeed, among other things, I would have us identify the negative quality of this experience as borne by consciousness in terms of the frustration of knowing that we lack the cultural resources for understanding the 'true' significance of our feelings of distress, and further, being made to recognise that our powers of reason are unable to reduce the hazardous uncertainty of the possible futures which await us. Moreover, I have gone so far as to suggest that where at the level of academic study there is a persistent conflict of interpretations with regard to the proper definition of anxiety, its precise causes and social distribution, then, in part, this may be understood as a consequence of the extent to which it is fundamental to anxiety that its 'objective' dimensions remain shrouded in obscurity. Accordingly, where there is always uncertainty in the lived experience of anxiety we may be certain that, as a topic for conceptual analysis, the 'reality' of this condition will remain open to debate.

Having identified anxiety as a problem of culture, I have also been concerned to highlight some of the social, economic and cultural processes which can be held responsible for making people more or less vulnerable to enter into this experience. Furthermore, insofar as our individual encounters with anxiety may be understood as an expression of the social conditions in which we are made to live, I have sought to present the task of coping as not so much a matter of personal disposition but, rather, as determined by the social opportunities and cultural resources which are made available to us for creating a positive meaning and sense of purpose for our lives. Accordingly, I have outlined a sociological conception of the problem of anxiety which emphasises the determining force of culture, economy and society upon the ways in which we negotiate the meaning of our personal circumstances so as to feel more or less 'in control' of the situations which evoke our feelings of distress. Moreover, where ultimately, sociology would have us identify our emotional and mental experience of the world as a product of society, I have outlined a range of critical questions for assessing the extent to which we might hope to achieve solutions to the problem of anxiety through a transformation of the social conditions which govern our individual choice of lifestyle.

I now turn my attention to the concept of risk and the contrasting ways in which this may be used to map the contours of our current 'age of anxiety'. Within the discourses of sociocultural theory the notion of risk now appears 'as one of the focal points of feelings of fear, anxiety and uncertainty' (Lupton 1999a: 12). Indeed, some even go so far as to identify the plethora of debates on risk in the public sphere of Western societies as the major cause and/or expression of the 'exaggerated' anxieties of our times (Furedi 1997). However, in the context of this book's more general sociological conception of the problem of anxiety, the concept of risk is understood as just *one* of the many symbolic forms of culture through which people might come to make sense of their feelings of distress; or rather, it may be that a small portion of our anxieties can be identified as aroused in connection with the self-perception of being 'at risk'. By no means am I inclined to represent and explain the majority of our anxieties in these terms. Indeed, where I have been concerned to outline a sociological conception of the problem of anxiety in contemporary societies, one of my aims is to equip the reader with a set of analytical tools which cast suspicion upon the contention that society is more anxious because it is more risk conscious.

In the next couple of chapters I offer a critical review of the contrasting ways in which the hermeneutics of risk might be used to interpret the causes and significance of anxiety in contemporary societies. I am concerned to highlight the conflicts of interpretation which characterise some of the most influential sociological accounts of the risk–anxiety relationship. Moreover, I will attempt to explain these differences not only as the result of disagreements over the meaning of 'risk', but also as a consequence of the extent to which the 'problem of anxiety' is liable to immerse us in the realms of speculation. First, I aim to highlight the potential for contrasting conceptions of risk to position us at different points along the tension between fear and anxiety; where on the one hand knowledge of risk may serve to allay anxiety by making clear the proper dimensions of an anticipated danger so that it can be faced as a manageable fear, on the other hand, this knowledge may be constructed so as to highlight the foreboding uncertainties of our future so that we become more vulnerable to the experience of anxiety. Second, I would alert the reader to the possibility of understanding the ongoing debate about the relationship between risk and anxiety as not only a consequence of the permutations of risk discourse and analysis, but also in terms of the extent to which the 'problem of anxiety' succeeds in defying our techniques of rationalisation; for it appears that where people are made vulnerable to experience anxiety there is always something which remains to be properly explained, organised and understood. Accordingly, where it is now becoming clear that there can be no final agreement on the magnitude of the risks we face and the extent to which a heightened sense of anxiety is a 'normal' and 'rational' response to the possible futures which await us, this may be recognised not only as a product of differences in political opinion about the reality of risk, but also as the inevitable consequence of the attempt to subject the experience of anxiety to our categories of rational understanding.

## ANXIETY IN A RISK SOCIETY

In the first section of this chapter I outline a brief history of the semantics of risk which highlights the growing complexity of this concept, as in recent years it has come to be used not only as a tool of actuarial procedure, but also as a means of debating the acceptability of political, economic and technological decisions made according to the mandate of calculative reason. Indeed, it is particularly in the context of the latter that I seek to explore the paradox that knowledge of risk can be used to both unsettle and reassure those seeking to plan for the future on the basis of the discernible patterns of events in our past. As the meaning of risk has become more subject to confusion and open to debate, then we find that where, on the one hand, this concept may appear to add weight to the certainty of our calculations of probable future outcomes, on the other, it may serve to accentuate the (potentially hazardous) uncertainty that comprises any attempt to apply the measures of reason to this task.

In the second section these paradoxes of risk are explored in terms of their significance for the experience of anxiety. In this context, I am particularly concerned to highlight the extent to which knowledge of risk may be conceived as standing at both ends of the tension between our knowledge and ignorance of fearful situations. Accordingly, I aim to explain how public debates on risk may be represented not only as a cause of anxiety, but also as a means of coping with the distress of this condition. As a matter of cultural interpretation (at least at the level of conceptual analysis), I consider both points of view to be equally plausible, given the varieties of meanings that can be made out of our knowledge of risk. However, in the context of sociology, writers tend to argue with the emphasis on either one side or the other: thus, where some would convince us that social representations of risk have become a favoured means by which people make an attempt at coping with their symptoms of emotional distress (Douglas 1992; Joffe 1999), others identify the public debates which revolve around these terms as a major cause of our anxieties (Beck 1992; Giddens 1991). These contrasting perspectives are compared not only with the aim of highlighting their opposing theoretical conceptions of the significance of 'risk consciousness' for the experience of anxiety, but also with the purpose of identifying some of the political implications of their favoured renditions of the risk–anxiety relationship.

In the final section I note that where we would adopt a selective point of view on the risk–anxiety relationship then, at least within the terms set by 'the risk debate' in social science, this may be interpreted not only as a political judgement upon the reality of risk but also (by implication) on the rationality of anxiety. Indeed, in this context, it appears that contrasting conceptions of the risk–anxiety relationship are politically motivated to persuade us towards a favoured perspective on the trustworthiness of expert opinion as well as the moral acceptability of the statistically improbable event of disaster. However, here I would emphasise that I am not concerned to present the reader with political reasons for privileging a particular interpretation of the cultural reality of our situation, rather, I am simply concerned to highlight the extent to which the risk debate is sustained by an inevitable conflict of interpretations.

## The semantic history of risk

The semantics of risk have a long history. Moreover, when looking back over the wide range of institutional contexts in which this concept has appeared as a means of expressing our knowledge of uncertainty, one is liable to come across the paradox that, where 'risk' is sometimes represented in terms of our confidence to discern future outcomes on the basis of our powers of calculative reason, on other occasions, it is used to emphasise the inexactitude of our predictions in face of the suspected 'wildness' (Bernstein 1998: 329–37) which remains hidden in the obscurity of future time. Knowledge of risk may serve to reinforce both our understanding and ignorance of the possible futures which await us. Indeed, I am particularly concerned to investigate the most recent developments in the social history of this concept in terms of the extent to which, depending upon the moral and political judgements which are cast upon the 'reality' in which we find ourselves, knowledge of risk may be used to construct different and opposing conceptions of the possible threat of danger as well as the social opportunities which are before us to achieve our preferred choice of lifestyle.

The etymology of the concept of risk is inconclusive but ultimately it may be derived from the Arabic word *risq* which means riches or good fortune (Skeat 1910). However, where there is also an attempt to recover its origins in the Greek word *rhiza*, meaning cliff, and the Latin *resegare,* meaning 'to cut off short', John Ayto suggests that risk may be understood to have its semantic roots embedded in a classical maritime vocabulary as a term invoking the perils of sailing too closely to inshore rocks (Ayto 1990). It is perhaps interesting to note that during the Middle Ages both of these possible meanings come together when the concept of risk is first adopted as a principle of maritime insurance. In this context, risk is used to refer to the assumption of acquisitive opportunities in face of potential misfortune and catastrophe.

Florence Edler de Roover claims that it was during the Commercial

Revolution (1275–1375) that Italian shipping merchants first began to use modern-style insurance contracts as a means of managing their business affairs (de Roover 1945). This period saw the emergence of a new type of business arrangement where, rather than travelling with their goods in order to secure a transaction, merchants could choose to stay at home and use a system of insurance loans as an incentive for shipowners to guarantee safe delivery of their cargo. Moreover, she notes that as these people acquired a greater confidence to invest in the probability of a successful venture, then it became possible to transfer the whole burden of risk to an indirectly attached third party as in a formal premium insurance contract. The earliest recorded examples of premium insurance contracts were drawn up in Palermo in 1350, however, it is possible that they were already in use before this date in the more important business centres of Florence and Pisa. Under the provisions of these contracts, the business relationship between insurer and the insured was reversed for the first time. Where under the system of sea loans, the insured party was obliged on safe arrival of his goods to pay a sum of money, the large part of which he had already received, by contrast, under the arrangement of premium insurance, the insurer, having agreed on a premium, received nothing in advance and was now obliged to pay out a sum of money even if the business venture ended in disaster.

In the context of insurance, the concept of risk may be identified as an abstract, transferable, symbolic representation of our relative confidence to assume control over the hazards of contingency (Ewald 1991). The communication of probabilities in terms of risk emerges in the wake of an increased technological and administrative capacity to reduce the apparent complexity and randomness of our world to a point where, on the basis of our accumulated knowledge of the regular pattern of occurrences in our past, it becomes possible to calculate the degree of uncertainty with which we might plan for the future. Such developments could only take place insofar as societies achieved a greater power to control the forces of nature (as well as their own citizens) whereby it became possible to place a measure of guarantee upon the predicted outcomes of investment decisions (de Roover 1945; Jackson 1989). Indeed, where the use of risk as a principle of insurance implies the successful establishment of a range of legal institutions, administrative practices, economic interests and technological appropriations which are basic to the development of modern capitalist societies, some would have us identify this with the origins of the social irruptions which ultimately gave rise to conditions of modernity (Luhmann 1991; Beck 1999: 50–2).

It was not until the nineteenth century that the technology of risk came to be systematically applied on a grand scale in the governance of society (Ewald 1991). As far as Britain is concerned Ian Hacking identifies the period between 1820 and 1840 as the time when an 'avalanche of numbers' first descended upon the ordering of human affairs (Hacking 1990; 1991). By the middle of the nineteenth century, statistical data on population trends had become an indispensable component of public debate on the ills of society. Indeed, among the 'moral scientists' of the day it was widely assumed that it was by the techniques of enumeration and classification that one might be able to discover a means of imposing more effective measures of control upon the 'deviant' elements of a population (Hacking 1990: 3). The first attempts to discover the statistical laws governing human social behaviour took place under the auspices of a moral and political project to reduce rates of crime, suicide, vagrancy, prostitution and disease.

By examining the history of these developments, Hacking's purpose is to identify the social conditions which inspired a major transformation in philosophical conceptions of 'objective knowledge' of reality. It appears that at the beginning of the nineteenth century, the intellectual community largely held to the view that chance played no part in the formation of social reality; rather, it was believed that the behaviour of society was ultimately determined by universal laws of nature. However, Hacking is concerned to argue that as new technologies of classification and enumeration were brought to bear upon the conditions of social life, the increasing amounts of statistical information that were gathered on the complexity and random elements of human behaviour enabled 'moral scientists' and philosophers to finally recognise the order of society as the product of laws of chance. The greater the attempt to impose measures of control upon the 'deviant' elements of a population, the more it became possible to identify the extent to which an 'ultimate indeterminism' lay behind the appearance of regularity in human affairs. Moreover, he understands this discovery to be heavily implicated in 'the most decisive conceptual event of the twentieth century', namely, that 'the world is not deterministic' (the past does not determine exactly what happens next), but rather, is part of 'a universe of absolute irreducible chance' (Hacking 1990: 1–10).

According to Bob Heyman and Mette Henriksen (1998), the historical process which Ian Hacking refers to as 'the taming of chance', that is, the inclusion of 'apparently chance or irregular events . . . under the control of natural or social law' (Hacking 1990: 10), is of vital importance for exploring the contemporary meaning of risk. They claim that it is in accordance with this greater knowledge of social indeterminacy that it becomes possible to recognise the 'reality' of risk as not so much a property of the world, but rather, a product of the ways we construct our knowledge of what must remain uncertain in the possible futures which await us. Understood as a 'simplifying heuristic' (Heyman 1998: 5) for guiding action in face of the irreducible indeterminism of the possible outcomes of complex social processes, the concept of risk may be identified not only as a means by which, with the maximum of certitude, we may attempt to predict and control the future, but also, as a way of constructing knowledge of the future which draws us face-to-face with the brute facts of our uncertainty.

Following Hacking, they emphasise that where the technologies for calculating probabilities are now more advanced than at any time in human history, along with more 'enlightened' information about the diverse range of factors which may influence the dynamics of future events in the natural and social world, we have acquired a greater knowledge of the dark areas of uncertainty which comprise our conceptions of the 'reality' of the risks we face. Where the discovery of the laws of probability which govern our collective social behaviour allow unprecedented opportunities to plan ahead according to the certainty of calculative reason, this also allows us to acquire a greater knowledge of the magnitude of indeterminacy which is contained in any attempt to predict the future. Heyman and Henriksen are concerned to highlight the extent to which calculations of risk encode only a partial knowledge of what the future might hold. Accordingly, while they understand conceptions of risk to be extremely valuable as a guide for decision and action in anticipation of possible future events, insofar as these require us to make simplifying assumptions about the outcomes of complex pseudo-random and indeterminate processes, then they would also alert us to the extent to which the assurances of risk analysis can sometimes be extremely misleading.

In the context of health care they note that where probability statements incorporating the language of risk may be used to highlight the chance of positive outcomes from medical interventions, on other occasions, this appears as a means of emphasising the elements of uncertainty and potential hazard associated with a particular procedure. For example, in their study of the communication of probabilities in prenatal genetic counselling Henriksen and Heyman (1998) found that:

> [A] woman may be told either that she has a probability of 1:100 of having a miscarriage through amniocentesis, or a probability of 99:100 of not suffering this adversity. Professionals may use the latter, more optimistic, descriptive device in order to encourage risk acceptance.
>
> (Heyman and Henriksen 1998: 28)

Moreover, Heyman notes that applications for research funding made to his local medical ethics committee tend to lay particular emphasis upon the extent to which such quantitative probability estimates may give a false impression of the accuracy of statistical calculations of risk (ibid.: 76). Accordingly, researchers may highlight the extent to which assessments of risk can only be achieved at the expense of a reduced conception of the complexity in real systems of cause and effect, particularly where these concern the vagaries of human behaviour. As far as the calculation of health risks is concerned, it is not only the case that it is often impossible to specify the full range of variables which may be implicated in the likelihood of an individual contracting a particular type of disease, but also that the ways in which people reflexively incorporate the knowledge of being labelled 'at risk' can be extremely unpredictable (ibid.: 71–80). Indeed, these writers place a particular emphasis upon the extent to which the unpredictability of patients' responses to being informed about risk can have both positive and negative outcomes as far as their long-term health is concerned (ibid.: 95–6): where some will respond to the threat of danger by taking every precautionary measure to enhance their chances of maximising their health, others may respond by adopting even more reckless forms of behaviour (ibid.: 71). Accordingly, the dissemination of knowledge about risk may actually reduce our capacity to predict the magnitude of its negative impact upon the ways in which a population experiences their health.

A similar focus upon the extent to which the technology of risk can be used both in support of the certainty of our predictions of future outcomes and as a means of revealing the ambiguity of the 'facts' on which these are based, is to be found in Peter Bernstein's (1998) historical account of the development of probabilistic thinking in the worlds of finance and commerce. Where on the one hand he celebrates the scientific progress and material prosperity which have been achieved under the guidance of modern techniques of risk management, on the other hand, he expresses alarm at the 'scary' uncertainty which is revealed by the organised attempt to plan for the future on the basis of patterns of events in our past. Once again, a particular emphasis is placed upon the extent to which our advanced technological ability to base decisions about the future on the details of our past is liable to increase the 'tension' between the assurances and uncertainties of risk. Bernstein argues that where the tools of risk analysis have become increasingly sophisticated, the more we learn about the 'discontinuities, irregularities and volatilities' of capital markets, the more likely it is that we will be made to question our ability to make investment plans on the basis of our accumulated knowledge of how economies performed in the past. Accordingly, where we come to recognise that 'surprise is endemic' in our history, Bernstein would have us question the extent to which risk management is either a science or an art; for the less we are able to rely upon the quantification of historical patterns of events as a means of predicting the future, the more we shall be left speculating on the basis of subjective leaps of faith (ibid.: 6–7).

According to François Ewald (1991; 1993), such developments may be understood to be heavily implicated in the contemporary bifurcation of the meaning of risk in Western societies. He argues that our advanced technological capacity for analysing social and economic processes in terms of risk is liable to exacerbate a debate on the acceptability of risk; for where the attempt to use the tools of calculative reason permits us to identify risks in every area of individual and collective decision, it may also be used to make people more alarmed about the precarious uncertainty of the relationships they hold towards the future. He suggests that it is particularly in relation to public debates about the potentially catastrophic consequences of modern industrial technologies that we can now identify some of the greatest divisions in the ways in which people mobilise their knowledge of risk. Where on the one hand governments and business corporations use expert assessments of risk so as to emphasise the extent to which the benefits of a particular technology far outweigh its costs and to convince 'the public' that every precautionary measure is in place so as to ensure their safety, on the other hand, some will seize upon the inevitable uncertainties of this knowledge so that where it remains possible to associate that technology with the (albeit highly remote) possibility of disaster, the risk will be deemed 'unacceptable'. Accordingly, Ewald notes that knowledge of risk may now be used on one side to highlight 'chance' and 'opportunity' and, on the other, to accentuate 'uncertainty' and 'danger'; where 'taking risks' in the spirit of enterprise tends to embrace its positive meaning, those that identify themselves as standing 'at risk', seek to draw attention to the potential for the future to visit us with danger. Indeed, he claims that where as a matter of everyday language one is now most likely to encounter the term being used as a synonym for 'danger', this testifies to the extent to which, during the last century, the massive expansion of the 'technology of risk' has *itself* exacerbated people's anxieties about the extent to which the industrial project of modernity may have damaging effects upon the health of populations and the natural environment.

While Mary Douglas presents us with a quite different way of understanding the causes of public anxiety (Douglas 1985; 1992; 1996; Douglas and Wildavsky 1982), she is also inclined to explain the popular usage of the term 'risk' as a synonym for 'danger' with reference to the impact of probabilistic thinking upon our culture and its rise to prominence as a source of legitimacy for future planning. However, she suggests that this should be understood not so much as a product of the extent to which expert risk analysis makes us more aware of the potentially hazardous uncertainties of our future but, rather, as a popular means of alerting others to the seriousness of our expressed anxieties by underlining them with the authority of science. Douglas claims that it is as a consequence of the valorisation of calculative reason and scientific procedure in our culture that people are most likely to adopt the vocabulary of risk when talking about their personal fears and anxieties. To simply identify oneself as being 'anxious' about a possible danger is hereby understood to have little impact upon the terms of public debate, but where a group declares themselves to be 'at risk', she argues that this is far more likely to exact a response from governments and other authoritative bodies of opinion, for the language of risk has the respected status of scientific rationality. She suggests:

> The probability theorists who developed risk assessment as a purely neutral, objective tool of analysis, must find it is much transformed as it moves into national and international politics. Though the public seems to be thinking politically in terms of comparative risks, the number-crunching does not matter; the idea of risk is transcribed simply as unacceptable danger. So 'risk' does not signify an all-round assessment of probable outcomes but becomes a stick for beating authority.
>
> (Douglas 1992: 39)

Accordingly, recent developments in the semantics of risk now lead the majority of commentators to emphasise the extent to which the meaning of this term has become more open to interpretation and more heavily disputed than at any other time in its history (Royal Society 1992; Ewald 1993; Adams 1995; Lupton 1999a). I would draw attention to the possibility of identifying a range of technological and cultural developments as each contributing something distinctive to this broad arena of debate. However, with the benefit of hindsight it may be impossible to conceive the dynamics of one source of dispute apart from its interrelationship with the whole gamut of controversy which comprises 'the risk debate' in Western societies.

In the first place, it is possible to understand public disputes surrounding the meaning of risk as a product of the extension and greater sophistication of the methods of calculative reason in the governance of society. Where the technology of risk was originally confined to the purposes of business insurance, engineering and natural science, it appears there was a far greater consensus among experts as to the 'realities' represented in their future projections and the accuracy of their techniques of analysis. When only a minority of the population have a vested interest in risk, it is far easier to conceive expert assessments as providing a value-free objective calculation of the probability of undesired consequences from our actions; the necessarily subjective leaps of prognostication which are contained within any attempt to measure uncertainty are far less likely to become politicised. However, with the extension of the technology of risk into every sphere of our social activity, it is not only the case that experts have become more alert to the fact that the simplifying assumptions of the heuristics of risk may provide us with a misleading conception of the social reality of human behaviour, but also that they have become more concerned with the extent to which this involves them in casting moral and political judgements upon the hidden 'wildness' in our future. Indeed, it seems writers such as Peter Bernstein are all too aware that, as the technology of risk is applied in ever more complex realms of speculation, then this itself becomes a means of alerting us to the extent to which the management of uncertainty may require us to make terrifying leaps of faith in the process of our decision-making (Bernstein 1998: 269–337). Where risk analysis serves to cast light upon the realms of possibility, it may also function to make us more cognisant of the dark reaches of our uncertainty. Moreover, in this context the management of risk may be revealed as coming more under the influence of qualitative opinion than a quantitative analysis of the 'hard facts' of life (Heyman 1998).

Second, it is with regard to the capacity for the technology of risk to function both to assure the certainty of our future predictions and as a means of placing them under suspicion, that writers such as François Ewald would draw our attention to the extent to which debates about the meaning of risk revolve around the contrasting sets of political values which govern people's judgements as to the acceptability of the decisions which are based on these terms. On this view, the more we come to think about our world in terms of risk, then the more likely it is that we shall witness conflicts of opinion with regard to what should be deemed an acceptable risk. He understands this to arise as a consequence of the fact that, where the tools of risk analysis may be used to reveal greater possibilities both in the realms of opportunity and potential catastrophe, they do not absolve us from having to make political and moral decisions as to what kinds of damage and loss are acceptable in light of the benefits which might be achieved. For Ewald it is particularly in the context of the potentially catastrophic consequences of industrial technologies and scientific experiments that the meaning of risk is now bound to political debates concerning the acceptability of technology and science. Here he conceives the technocratic decisions which are made on the basis of risk analysis to have the effect of dividing public opinion on the meaning of risk to the point where this term can no longer be evoked simply to refer to the 'objective' measure of probable outcomes, but rather, becomes inextricably entwined with the conflicting political judgements which are cast upon the acceptability of the possible dangers associated with polluting technologies and the science of genetics. Ewald writes:

> Even if technology enables us to know the risk, it cannot eliminate or solve the problem of having to choose whether or not to accept the risk. As risk assessment specialists clearly state, there is no such thing as risk in itself. The effective reality of a risk, that which 'creates' the risk, is the contestation to which it may give rise. This is not to say that there are no objective risks, that the launching of a giant oil tanker, an airplane flight, or the construction of a nuclear power plant or chemical factory does not carry objective risks. The problem resides not in the existence of these risks in the abstract, but in the fact of their acceptance by a population . . . the bigger the objective risk (for example, one on the scale of a catastrophe), the more dependent its reality is on a system of values.
>
> (1993: 225)

Third, the work of writers such as Mary Douglas, among other things, seeks to alert us to the extent to which the politicisation of risk involves this concept in forms of discourse which take place outside the institutional domain of expert analysis. Where this term comes to be used exclusively as a means of evoking the threat of danger or as a blaming device in the realms of public dispute, she emphasises the extent to which the meaning of risk may be far removed from the influence of probabilistic thinking; where 'risk' means 'danger', one should certainly not presume that this has any *direct* connection to disputes in the context of actuarial procedure. While the rhetoric of risk may be understood to resonate with the authority of science, it may be used with no thought of science in mind. That is not to say that people may not identify certain types of science and technology as a possible cause of their anxieties but, rather, it is to emphasise the extent to which their feelings of distress may have little to do with the course of probabilistic thinking and its capacity to fuel the tension between the assurances and uncertainties of risk. For Douglas, the labelling of certain activities and possible future events as 'risk' is more a matter of cultural disposition than a product of statistical calculation. Of course, if it were not for the privileged status of scientific rationality in our culture, it is doubtful that we would have acquired this everyday language of risk, however, on this view, it is the selective types of danger which come to be labelled in these terms which require sociological explanation.

At this point in my discussion, I am simply concerned to highlight the extent to which the concept of risk may be used in a variety of ways and with quite different ends in mind. Where on the one hand, knowledge about risk implies certainty of calculation, controlled planning and assured prognosis, on the other, it may serve to give weight to our uncertainty and do no more than expose the haphazard indeterminacy of our fate. Moreover, where an emphasis on one side may be for the sake of acquisition, chance and progress, on the other, it could be with the purpose of alerting us to our vulnerability to damage, loss and misfortune. In the social history of this concept it is possible to identify a range of developments which contribute to present disagreements and confusions surrounding the 'reality' of risk and the extent to which we should identify our future with danger. While the 'risk debate' may be conceived in part as a direct result of the greater sophistication and social application of our techniques of calculative reason, we should recognise it is comprised of moral judgements and political values which defy analysis in these terms. Furthermore, where it is possible to understand the involvement of risk within conflicts of political opinion as a direct product of the extent to which calculations of risk involve us in commitments of value, we should be alert to the fact that, at the level of everyday language, conflicting views on risk may be more an expression of value than a result of a population's commitment to the disciplines of actuarial procedure. However, ultimately it may be impossible to distinguish differences of opinion at one level of discourse as entirely separable from the dynamics of the other.

## The risk–anxiety relationship: theoretical points of view

How might we conceive of the relationship between knowledge about risk and the experience of anxiety? Certainly, the semantic histories of the concepts of risk and anxiety should alert us to the likelihood of there being a wide range of possible answers to this question. However, for the sake of clarity, and in following my emphasis upon the extent to which the experience of anxiety may be understood to thrive upon the tension between our knowledge and ignorance of fearful situations, I would highlight two basic and contrasting ways in which we might conceive of the moderating force of 'risk consciousness' upon our vulnerability to anxiety.

In the first place, where knowledge of risk may do no more than make us aware of possible futures which contain unknown quantities of danger, it can certainly be represented as a possible cause of anxiety. On this view, the significance of 'risk consciousness' for anxiety may be understood to reside in its potential to make us more cognisant of the foreboding obscurity of future time. Where writers conceive knowledge of risk as a cause of anxiety, an emphasis tends to be placed upon the capacity for the uncertainties of risk to inscribe our conceptions of the future with the marks of menace, possible pain and hidden danger; to be made 'risk conscious' is to acquire a greater awareness of how hazardous our ignorance of the future can be.

By contrast, insofar as knowledge of risk may be conceived as a means of making certain our understanding of future possibilities, its significance for anxiety may be understood to consist more in terms of its capacity to be used as a resource for coping, than in its propensity to stand among the causes of this condition. In this context, an emphasis may be placed upon the ways in which 'risk consciousness' serves to allow people to objectify the proper dimensions of an anticipated danger so that it becomes clear how they should live and what they must do in order to keep themselves out of harm's way. It is with regard to the utility of this concept for casting light upon the obscurity of a suspiciously hazardous future that knowledge of risk may help us to control the effects of anxiety by providing us with a clear focus for our fears. Accordingly, it is with an interest in the ways in which people attempt to assure themselves of the 'reality' of dangers to be faced, challenged and overcome that some would have us interpret 'risk consciousness' more as a response to anxiety than its cause.

Knowledge of risk may be identified as standing at both ends of the tension between our knowledge and ignorance of fearful situations. In the works of Ulrich Beck (1992; 1995; 1997; 1998; 1999) and Anthony Giddens (1990; 1991; 1998) we find the greater emphasis being placed upon knowledge of risk as the cause of anxiety, while by contrast, Mary Douglas (1985; 1992; Douglas and Wildavsky 1982) and Hélène Joffe (1999) are more interested to explore the cultural implications of the interrelationship between anxiety, risk and coping. Moreover, according to their preferred points of emphasis these theorists present us with a range of quite different readings of the politics of a society in which people are (allegedly) becoming more 'risk conscious'. I will outline each perspective in turn. However, for the purposes of this chapter I am not concerned to question the accuracy of these theorists' conflicting interpretations of the risk–anxiety relationship, and nor would I argue for any particular point of view on the emergent politics of a 'risk society'; rather, I would simply place an emphasis upon the extent to which, given the semantic history of risk and the peculiar phenomena of the experience of anxiety, a conflict of interpretations is precisely what we should come to expect.

## Risk, endangerment and anxiety

Anthony Giddens and Ulrich Beck have focused exclusively upon the potential for a greater knowledge of risk to make us feel more insecure about our place in society and arouse our anxieties with regard to the possibly catastrophic futures which await us.' Both conceive an important role for the mass media in the cultivation of a type of 'risk consciousness' which they understand to increase levels of existential doubt among the populations of Western societies as they become more cognisant of a future of possible hazard and hidden danger (Giddens 1991: 1–34; Beck 1992: 22–4). For these theorists the social and political significance of 'risk consciousness' should be identified in terms of the extent to which a greater public knowledge of risk is liable to make us morbidly preoccupied with our future safety and fuels public debates on the benefits of modern technology and the morality of science.

Giddens provides us with a general conception of the erosion of our 'ontological security' as we become aware of the 'high-consequence risks' of a 'late modern' society. He suggests that now more than ever, we are inclined to negotiate our futures with a calculative attitude towards the future which consciously weighs up the chance of self-fulfilment with the risk of endangerment (Giddens 1991: 28). However, for Giddens, knowledge of risk has little to do with placing confidence in the predictive power of calculative reason but, rather, with the extent to which the limits of rationalisation are liable to arouse in us a sense of foreboding. 'Risk consciousness' is hereby understood to be heavily implicated within the development of existential doubts and the self-perception of being 'in danger'. He suggests that public debates about the safety of public transport, health risks, food scares, environmental pollution, economic insecurity, crime and the threat of war all combine to create a 'generalised climate of risk' which for most people becomes 'a source of unspecific anxieties' (ibid.: 109–43, 181–208). On this view it is alleged that a 'reflexive' consciousness of risk 'creates a moral disquiet that individuals can never fully overcome' (ibid.: 185).

Beck's discussion shares many of the themes in Giddens' analysis of our present 'culture of risk', however, he is particularly interested to explore the extent to which the anxiety aroused by the 'manufactured uncertainty' of public debates on hazard may serve as a critical movement for the political reform of industrial societies. He suggests that where populations acquire a greater knowledge of the potentially catastrophic hazards of modern (nuclear and chemical) technology and the possibly disastrous 'side-effects' of scientific experiments, then we are likely to witness the emergence of 'a social epoch in which solidarity from anxiety becomes a political force' for directing the future course of development within industrial modernity (Beck 1992: 49). Indeed, his more recent attempts at describing the contours of political debate in a 'world risk society' may be understood to be largely inspired by the suggestion that we are living in an age where 'the social power of anxiety' (ibid.) becomes a major preoccupation for governments and industries who preside over the technological colonisation of our future (Beck 1997; 1998; 1999). More so than Giddens, Beck's analysis focuses upon the potential radicalism of the risk–anxiety relationship; he has a major interest in the extent to which this might serve as the inspiration for an emancipatory politics which seeks to bring a halt to the development and implementation of technologies which court the risk of global environmental catastrophe.

For both of these theorists the significance of public knowledge of risk lies in the extent to which it makes us more uncertain about the future. Where our minds are filled with thoughts of risk, then we are understood to acquire an amplified sense of doubt with regard to our personal ability to live in safety. The social significance of 'risk consciousness' resides in its capacity to make us anxiously preoccupied with maximising our powers of control over the course of our destiny; allegedly, it has the effect of making us radically call into question how we should live and what we must do in order to keep ourselves from harm's way. Indeed, 'risk consciousness' is held to open up the terms of public debate on the possible futures which await us. Ulrich Beck goes so far as to identify this with a vanguard movement for the 'reinvention' of politics (Beck 1997; 1999). He invests considerable hope in the possibility that 'the introduction of insecurity into our thought and deeds may help to achieve the reduction of objectives, slowness, revisability and ability to learn, the care, consideration, tolerance and irony that are necessary for a change to a new modernity' (Beck 1997: 168).

### Anxiety, risk and coping

In the works of Mary Douglas (1985; 1992; 1996; Douglas and Wildavsky 1982) and Hélène Joffe (1999) we find an opposing interpretation of the cultural significance of risk. These writers are concerned with the possibilities for people to use their knowledge of risk as a means of coping with their anxiety and putting paid to existential doubts. Following the terms of analysis developed in earlier chapters of this book, I understand them to be interested to explore the ways in which 'risk consciousness' functions to translate the uncertainties of anxiety into the sure knowledge of fear. Their theories are inspired by a tradition of Durkheimian sociology which leads them to understand our current preoccupation with risk as not so much a consequence of the extent to which we have acquired a calculative attitude towards our future, but rather, as a result of our moral commitments towards different forms of social solidarity. Moreover, when considering political disputes on risk, this leads them to focus more upon the extent to which people use the language of risk in an effort to close off the terms of public debate in the direction of their favoured point of view. They are not so much impressed by the possibility that 'risk consciousness' may cause us to question and criticise our accepted understandings of the world but, rather, with the extent to which this serves to shore up our convictions as to how we should live and what we should do in order to maintain our preferred way of life.

Mary Douglas understands all knowledge of self and society to be shaped according to our basic human need to establish moral rules for regulating our social relationships and maintaining the moral order of society. Throughout her career she has consistently sought 'to treat cultural categories as the cognitive containers in which social interests are defined and classified, argued and negotiated, and fought out' (Douglas 1982: 12). She is particularly concerned to trace the cultural boundaries which demarcate our systems of meaning and classification so as to understand the ways in which these function to maintain relations of social solidarity. On this view, the cultural significance of risk lies in the extent to which it is used to endow the world with moral meaning and to defend our sense of order and justice. Above all else, she would have us identify the language of risk as a means of casting blame on 'others' who are perceived to represent a threat to 'our' health and livelihood.

Douglas understands contemporary anxieties in terms of Durkheimian anomie and she interprets public disputes about risk as collective attempts to impose a greater sense of moral order upon society. Accordingly, where certain sections of the populations of Western societies are becoming more preoccupied with the risk of environmental disaster, she interprets this not so much as a consequence of the escalating threat of danger, but rather as a result of the ways in which the erosion of social solidarity among marginalised groups inspires them to adopt ecological catastrophism as a means of protecting their preferred way of life (Douglas and Wildavsky 1982; Dake and Wildavsky 1990). Douglas would alert us to the possibility of understanding cultural representations of the threat of disaster as a means by which people cope with the anxiety of anomie; the perceived risk of imminent disaster serves to unite disparate individuals around a common cause, and the shared focus on extreme danger functions to censure the egoistic impulse towards disunity. She suggests that in a secular culture in which science has acquired the 'sacred' authority of traditional forms of religion, the concept of 'nature' has replaced the idea of 'God'. Where in the past, marginalised groups would invoke the 'wrath of God' on behalf of their feelings of resentment towards central authorities, in our society 'the backlash of nature' serves a similar purpose; the threat of ecological disaster has become a source of moral legitimation for groups excluded from and opposed to the establishment (Douglas and Wildavsky 1982; Douglas 1992) .

For Douglas and colleagues working under the banner of 'Cultural Theory' (Thompson *et al.* 1990; Schwarz and Thompson 1990; Dake and Wildavsky 1990; Dake 1991, 1992), we should understand public disputes on risk as not so much to do with disagreements over the accuracy of 'objective' calculations of future possibilities but, rather, as a reflection of the cultural dispositions of different groups to entrust themselves to a ('theological') perspective on nature and society which conforms to their prior experiences of social solidarity. On this view, when it comes to deciding which risks are most worrisome and which are best left ignored, our choice is invariably settled by the quality of our moral commitments towards favoured institutions. There is no objective value-neutral means of assessing the reality of risk, rather, what we come to believe about the magnitude of the dangers we face is, in the last instance, determined by a qualitative decision to entrust ourselves to a vision of the future which conforms to the morality of our ideal way of life. Accordingly, in the social contexts of everyday life, the language of risk is conceived as a means by which people endeavour to make clear the 'truth' about how we should live and what we must do. Where a population displays signs of 'risk consciousness', we should interpret this not so much as a sign of existential doubt and a disposition to question the meaning of the world but, rather, as an attempt to articulate and defend a preferred point of view on reality. Knowledge of risk is not so much involved in creating uncertainty and evoking anxiety; rather, it functions socially as a means of allaying the distress of uneasy suspense by providing us with a clear focus for our fears. Moreover, where we may be convinced of the true 'reality' of future hazards, then the language of risk may serve as a 'forensic resource' for casting blame on those who are perceived to have placed us in danger.

More recently, Hélène Joffe (1999) has outlined a social psychological theory to explain this behaviour. She draws on a number of sources such as Kleinian psycho-dynamic theory (Klein 1929; 1946), attribution theory (Heider 1958; Kelley 1973; Ross 1977), 'optimistic bias' research (Weinstein 1980; 1982; 1987) and (principally) Serge Moscovici's work on social representations (Farr and Moscovici 1984), in order to detail an analytical framework for investigating a common human response to the risk of danger, namely: 'not me, not my group, others are to blame' (Joffe 1999: 1). She maintains that in times of crisis, the most common psychic response is to blame 'others' who are 'outside' one's group for bringing chaos into the world. Following Douglas (1992), she suggests that all cultures use scapegoating as a means of coping with the perceived threat of danger and the language of risk is ideally suited for this purpose. Moreover, she argues that such a response also serves to build up feelings of personal invulnerability to the danger; for it is not only the case that 'others' are to blame, but also the risk is most likely to be portrayed as 'their' problem, not 'ours'.

Joffe refers us to her cross-cultural studies of group reactions to the risk of contracting HIV/AIDS. In this context, she notes that when asked to express personal opinions on AIDS, regardless of their particular cultural background, people commonly seek to 'split' themselves away from the threat of danger by focusing their blame upon distant 'others' who are perceived to have unleashed disorder upon the world. She found that where the majority of South Africans tend to blame the 'sinful' practices of Western populations for the spread of AIDS, most British people are inclined to identify the origins of the disease in the 'alien' sexual practices of African tribes (Joffe 1999: 40–2). In each instance, respondents are inclined to distance their own group from the source of the disease and blame distant 'others' for creating the risk of danger. Accordingly, Joffe argues that as a basic response to crisis and hazard, humans are psychically driven to protect the sanctity of their own 'in-group' identity, and further, are liable to display a basic emotional impulse to perceive themselves as not only personally exempt from blame, but also, invulnerable to harm. On this view the social representation of risk functions not only as a means of legitimating 'our' preferred rendition of the 'truth' about the reality in which we find ourselves, but also, as a defence mechanism against anxiety in which the threat of AIDS is more likely to be seen as a problem for 'others' who are not like 'us'.

For Douglas and Joffe, the political significance of 'risk consciousness' should most certainly not be identified in terms of its inspiration for critical reflexivity, rather, our cultural preoccupation with risk should be interpreted as a sign of people's closed mindedness and resistance to change (Douglas 1996: 161–92; Joffe 1999: 126–45). On this view, the politics of risk holds no prospect of opening up the public sphere to the terms of critical debate, rather, it is comprised of mutually antagonistic worldviews which offer no space for shared understanding and ethical compromise. Indeed, the language of risk is understood to work as a defence against anxiety insofar as it serves to enable people to distance themselves from self-doubt and convince them of the moral virtue of their favoured point of view on reality. The significance of risk for the task of coping lies in the extent to which it serves to translate the uncertainties of anxiety into the sure knowledge of fear. Accordingly, for Douglas and Joffe, where large numbers of people are committed to negotiating the meaning of their futures in terms of risk, then we should anticipate that they will have entrenched opinions with regard to how we should think and what we should do so as to make secure our preferred way of life.

## The 'reality' of risk and the rationality of anxiety

These contrasting conceptions of the risk–anxiety relationship have attracted widespread debate throughout the social sciences. However, the provocation of these theorists is generally understood to reside not so much in what they have to say about anxiety, but rather, in their contrasting assessments of the 'reality' of risk (Adams 1995; Lupton 1999a; 1999b; Crook 1999). In particular, it is with reference to the political points of view which writers such as Ulrich Beck and Mary Douglas cast upon public reactions to the hazards of industrial technologies and the risk of ecological catastrophe that the terms of debate have been set. Where Beck's 'risk society' thesis is inspired by the view that Western civilisation is faced with the very real threat of 'self-annihilation', Douglas' cultural anthropology is generally understood to cast doubt upon such an apocalyptic scenario.

Where in Douglas' analysis our individual perceptions of risk are understood to be heavily influenced by the quality of our prior commitments to different types of social organisation, then she would encourage us to interpret 'moral panics' over the safety of our natural environment not so much as a reasonable response to the 'reality' of danger, but rather, as an emotional/cultural reaction to the social experience of marginalisation. Such a perspective suggests that we should understand people's expressed views on risk as only marginally (if at all) concerned with statistical calculations of the costs and benefits of industrial technologies and, rather, place the greater emphasis upon the extent to which public debates on risk are 'surrogate for other social and ideological concerns' (Slovic 1987: 285). Accordingly, we are encouraged to consider the anxieties of environmental social movements to be exaggerated as a consequence of the extent to which the poverty of their experience of social solidarity disposes them to adopt a worldview which is inclined towards catastrophism (Douglas and Wildavsky 1982).

The emphasis of Mary Douglas and the proponents of Cultural Theory has found widespread appeal among those seeking to denounce public anxieties surrounding risks to our health and environment as no more than ideological scaremongering. As Deborah Lupton observes: 'Douglas' writings are frequently interpreted as implying that lay perceptions of risk involve inaccuracies and errors of judgement because of the contaminating influence of social and cultural processes' (1999a: 56). Accordingly, Frank Furedi notes the merits of her theory for exposing public concerns with risk as a social construction which is more the result of the growth of individualism and breakdown of community than a proportional response to the reality of danger (Furedi 1997: 8). On this view, many of the fears expressed in the mass media surrounding the safety of our foods, the risks of new technologies and dangers to our children are interpreted as a sign of 'society's loss of nerve' and 'the morality of low expectation' (ibid.: 45–71). Furedi repeatedly refers us to statistics gathered on the risk of accidental death and injury in connection with new health technologies and the recorded numbers of deaths resulting from toxins in our food in order to suggest that where there is only a highly remote possibility that we will come to grief as a result of taking the contraceptive pill or eating British beef, then we should understand 'the public' to be panicking unnecessarily about selective risks which are highly unlikely to cause them any harm. Thus, he decries the 'moral panics' surrounding the hazards of technology and the safety of the environment for the extent to which they contribute to a pessimistic view of our humanity, as though it were morally incapable of applying its technology towards self-improvement. Indeed, he is concerned to blame the 'culture of fear' for resigning us to a future in which the 'worship of safety' obstructs the development of 'progress' insofar as this thrives upon our ability to take creative risks.

However, such arguments are unlikely to dissuade Ulrich Beck from the view that we are living on the brink of self-annihilation, and that a heightened state of anxiety is a right and proper response to this 'fact'. For Beck, actuarial guarantees of safety are irrelevant in light of the knowledge that there are still rare occasions where the statistically improbable event of disaster takes place. He argues that in the aftermath of events such as 'Chernobyl' we have objective proof of the fact that the technologies of industrial modernity may have catastrophic 'side-effects' of potentially global proportions. Against those who refer us to the cultural relativity of hazard perception so as to represent his apocalyptic warnings as an hysterical overreaction to the unlikely event of ecological disaster, he urges us to consider 'Chernobyl' as a terrible sign of the real 'truth' of our situation, which is that 'we are caught in the trap the world has become' (Beck 1995: 74–110).

It is the political and moral significance which he attaches to the statistically improbable event of catastrophe which is important here. As far as Beck is concerned, the mere fact that we have even the slightest reason to believe in the possibility that such nightmare scenarios may one day become 'real-life' events justifies the response of high anxiety. Indeed, in retrospect, the twentieth century provides us with a number of terrifying examples of occasions where the lives of large numbers of people were devastated by disasters, which according to the terms of risk analysis would always be calculated as extremely remote possibilities; history teaches that there are no ultimate guarantees of safety. Following François Ewald, Beck's thesis is inspired by the view that with regard to the possible 'mega-hazards' of nuclear and chemical technologies, the statistically improbable event of disaster is morally unacceptable.

The longer it continues, the more patently clear it becomes that the debate between the so-called 'realist' and 'social constructivist' conceptions of risk cannot be resolved with any simple reference to undisputed bodies of 'objective' evidence. As I have emphasised in earlier sections of this chapter, as far as the heuristics of risk are concerned, those who weigh up the facts of our uncertainty are always committed to expressing a culturally relative point of view. In this context, it is increasingly apparent that there are no 'facts' aside from political and moral judgements which are cast upon the possible futures which await us. Indeed, even the Royal Society, which at one time appeared to be firmly committed to the view that one could maintain a clear distinction between 'objective' and perceived risk (Royal Society 1983), now openly acknowledges that:

> the view that a separation can be maintained between 'objective' risk and 'subjective' or perceived risk has come under increasing attack, to the extent that it is no longer a mainstream position . . . assessments of risk, whether they are based upon individual attitudes, the wider beliefs within a culture, or on the models of mathematical risk assessment, necessarily depend upon human judgement.
>
> (Royal Society 1992: 89–90)

This is openly acknowledged by both Ulrich Beck and Mary Douglas. Indeed, in the context of risk management the significance of their works is generally recognised in terms of their critical concern to expose the determining force of cultural values upon professional and lay opinions about risk (ibid.: 89–134; Adams 1995). However, we still find them arguing for the greater 'objectivity' of their own favoured points of view (Douglas 1996: 161–92; Beck 1995: 73–110). For example, despite her insistence that all knowledge of risk is subject to the mediating force of cultural bias, we find Mary Douglas arguing that 'the benefit of cultural theory is to provide distance and objectivity' (Douglas 1996: 175). It seems surprisingly easy for her to leave the institutional and political biases of Cultural Theory outside the domain of analytical debate. Similarly, while we find Ulrich Beck openly acknowledging that 'hazards are subject to historico-cultural perceptions and assessments which vary from country to country, from group to group, from one period to another' (Beck 1995: 91), and that the rationality of risk perception is always open to social definition (Beck 1992: 59), he still devotes the greater part of his discussion to the work of convincing us that society is faced with the very real threat of self-annihilation.

As far as John Adams is concerned, where these writers expose the cultural construction of risk perception only to argue for the superior rationality of their favoured points of view, then they 'spectacularly miss the point of all their preceding argument and analysis' (Adams 1995: 194). Moreover, he explains this as a refusal to face up to the fact that all perceptions of risk take place from positions of uncertainty. Accordingly, he understands them to 'crave a certainty that the physical scientists and their own theories tell them they can never have' (ibid.). However, I prefer to explain this in terms of their overriding political ambitions. I suggest that Beck and Douglas are not so much concerned to investigate the ways in which people acquire and create knowledge of 'hazards' as 'risks', but are more interested to cast 'the risk debate' in political perspective. Accordingly, on behalf of the polemical orientation of their theories, they would both have the rhetoric of objectivity on their side (Wilkinson 2001). In both instances, a critical focus on the cultural construction of risk is used more to expose the ideological interests of their opponents' views than it is to reflect upon the significance of their own institutional biases for the ways they represent 'the risk debate' to their readers.

Where the 'reality' of risk is disputed, we also find writers concerned to express views on the rationality of anxiety. The basic premise that we are living in times of high anxiety is not in question here, rather, it is the justification of the response of anxiety which is open to debate. According to the political judgements which they cast upon the magnitude of the risks we face, these writers seek to convince us that they possess the analytical keys for interpreting the greater 'truth' about the anxieties of contemporary society. Here, I would simply place an emphasis upon the extent to which it is only as a result of our own political commitments to one side or the other of a discursive struggle for definition that we shall find ourselves persuaded to adopt any particular point of view on these matters (Freudenberg and Pastor 1992).

## Conclusion

In this chapter I have highlighted some of the contrasting ways in which the hermeneutics of risk may be used to interpret the cultural significance of anxiety. I have been particularly concerned to emphasise the extent to which recent developments within the semantics of risk present us with the possibility of recognising 'information' expressed in these terms as standing at both ends of the tension between our knowledge and ignorance of fearful situations. Accordingly, where on the one hand 'risk consciousness', by its potential to alert us to the foreboding obscurity of our situation, may be interpreted as a cause of anxiety, on the other, where this is understood to cast light upon the 'real' object of our fears, it may be conceived to function more for the task of coping.

Moreover, I have emphasised the extent to which these contrasting interpretations of the risk–anxiety relationship are wedded to conflicting views on the 'reality' of the risks we face. In this context, I would have us recognise the extent to which (at least at the level of conceptual analysis), our preference for one interpretation as superior to the other cannot be defended on the basis of an appeal to the undisputed 'facts' about the risks we face but, rather, this implies a political point of view on the possible futures which await us and the kinds of lifestyle we would lead. Here my purpose is not to develop any detailed analysis of the political issues at stake, nor am I motivated to express a clear preference for one side or another of 'the risk debate', rather, I am simply concerned to highlight the extent to which opposing political interests are liable to sustain conflicting interpretations of the significance of 'risk consciousness' for the experience of anxiety. In this chapter I have focused primarily upon the ways in which the permutations of risk analysis and debate provide us with quite different ways of interpreting the anxiety of our times and its justification as a response to the perceived threat of danger. Where these issues will feature once more as a major theme in the following chapter, I will also be concerned to focus in more detail on some of the possible ways in which the problem of anxiety, in its own terms, may be conceived as a vital spur to the ongoing debate on risk.

# 5

## A speculative age

So far my account of the relationship between 'risk consciousness' and anxiety has been conducted almost exclusively at the level of conceptual analysis. In this context, I have devoted the large part of my discussion to describing some of the ways in which debates surrounding the meaning and 'reality' of risk may be used to construct opposing theoretical accounts of the significance of public debates on risk for the experience of anxiety. Moreover, I have made an attempt to explain how developments within the technology of risk, as well as opposing political points of view on the 'reality' of the hazards we face, are involved in conflicting interpretations of the risk–anxiety relationship. Indeed, I have sought to highlight the extent to which the political commitments of writers such as Ulrich Beck and Mary Douglas may be influencing their respective choices of emphasis on risk as either the cause of anxiety, or alternatively, as a symbolic resource for coping with this condition.

With reference to the problem of anxiety as conceived in earlier chapters of this book, I have been particularly concerned to highlight the extent to which it is possible to recognise 'risk consciousness' as standing at both ends of the tension between our knowledge and ignorance of fearful situations. In what follows, I seek to develop my critical account of 'the risk debate' in the social sciences with the main purpose of emphasising the extent to which all attempts at distinguishing the significance of 'risk consciousness' for the experience of anxiety are liable to enter into the realms of speculation. Indeed, I would argue that there will always be a range of conflicting interpretations when it comes to determining the ways in which our anxieties may be related to knowledge about the risks we face. So far I have noted the extent to which contrasting accounts of the risk–anxiety relationship are sustained in relation to political disagreements over the meaning of risk, however, here I shall ultimately be concerned to consider the extent to which it may be due to the peculiarity of the condition of anxiety itself that, so long as this remains part of our experience of everyday life, we should expect there to be no final agreement upon its precise causes, or for that matter, how we might best cope under the burden of its distressing affects.

In addition to this, and as a means of elaborating upon the theme of speculation, a large part of my discussion will also be devoted to exploring some of the analytical problems involved in determining how people may be thinking and *feeling* in relation to debates on risk in the public sphere of Western societies. A maxim attributed to Freud states: 'All that matters is love and work'; and in previous chapters I have noted that there is a considerable amount of empirical evidence to suggest that the social conditions of work and the quality of our relationships of emotional dependency are what matter most in relation to our vulnerability to anxiety. With this in mind, I have argued that if we were to look for some sociologically 'objective' indicators of the overall prevalence of this condition in society then, among other things, we might consider the degree of income distribution and the extent of relative poverty as well as the rates of unemployment and divorce to serve this purpose. In the context of stress research, it is with reference to the clearly observable and/or consistently expressed negative impact of such processes and events upon our bodies and minds that they are recognised as most significant for revealing the social distribution of anxiety. However, by contrast I would emphasise the extent to which the possible associations between the terms of public sphere debate and the ways in which people experience their anxieties can only be sustained as a matter of theoretical speculation. Certainly, it is the case that there is no clearly demonstrable link between the majority of publicly debated issues on risk and aetiologically significant experiences of anxiety. Indeed, as a number of writers suggest, the types of anxiety that are possibly associated with 'risk consciousness' are most likely to be 'free-floating', 'diffuse' and 'unspecific' (Furedi 1997; Giddens 1991); in accepting its (alleged) existence we are required to make an imaginative leap into 'a theoretically determined consciousness of reality' (Beck 1992: 73).

It is particularly with regard to public issues which are only made 'present' to our field of concern through the media of television, radio and newspapers that sociologists have begun to speculate upon the significance of 'risk consciousness' for our current 'age of anxiety'. Accordingly, the majority of sociological debates on the relationship between risk and anxiety concern public issues and social problems which only have an occasional presence in our mass media as topics of 'news', and outside this context are unlikely to appear among our most immediate concerns of everyday life. By examining this point in more detail I intend not only to develop my emphasis upon the conflict of interpretations surrounding the significance of 'risk consciousness' for anxiety, but further explore the significance of the condition of anxiety itself for ensuring that these discursive struggles of definition remain a topic of sociological concern. Indeed, I am inclined to suggest that the problem of anxiety on its own terms lends legitimacy to this particular field of debate; for so long as people are driven to seek solutions to the problem of anxiety, then we may anticipate that there will always be work for the 'sociological imagination' in identifying public issues to make sense of their 'personal troubles of milieu' (Mills 1959: 8).

The first three sections explore the interrelationship between media, risk and anxiety. Here I focus most of my attention upon the task of interpreting the significance of the contents of news media messages on risk for the ways in which people perceive and experience knowledge about 'hazards'. In this context, by exposing the conflict of interpretations which arises in the attempt to identify media representations of risk as representative of dominant attitudes in society, I would emphasise that speculation reigns in all attempts to establish the social reality of a 'risk society' on the basis of the evidence of discourses in the realms of public debate. In the final section, while reflecting upon the extent to which the problem of anxiety may be held to consist in our capacity for speculation, I outline some of the possible ways in which this is liable to have a continuing impact upon sociological endeavours to determine the cultural significance of risk consciousness in our times.

## A mediated 'shadow kingdom'

Ulrich Beck identifies a key role for mass media in the development and spread of 'risk consciousness', for he emphasises that in most instances, the particular risks that may be associated with the threat of 'self-annihilation', such as radioactivity, toxins and pollutants 'evade human perceptive abilities' (Beck 1992: 22). He argues that 'what eludes sensory perception only becomes socially available to "experience" in media pictures and reports'

(Beck 1995: 100). Accordingly, Beck suggests that the 'risk society' may be thought of as a kind of 'shadow kingdom' where the presence of danger always remains obscured; we are heavily dependent upon mass media to bring the 'real' horrors of our situation to light.

For most people, the majority of hazards debated in the context of the 'risk discourse' of social science may only be apprehended in terms of their symbolic representation in mass media. Generally speaking, the first, and sometimes the *only* time and place where we come into contact with issues such as the hazards of new genetic technologies and the threat of ecological disaster, is when we read our newspapers and watch television news. For many researchers, when considering why and how people become preoccupied with selective types of unusual risks while apparently giving little thought to commonplace hazards which are more likely to cause them harm, it seems obvious to look to the media for an explanation (Mazur 1981; Singer and Endreny 1987; Pilisuk and Acredolo 1988; Stallings 1990; Hornig 1990; 1992; Coleman 1993; Spencer and Triche 1994; Powell and Leiss 1997; Furedi 1997; Anderson 1997; Eldridge 1999). For instance, Roger and Jeanne Kasperson are now typical in placing a particular emphasis upon the extent to which not only the volume of media messages on risk, but also the (usually melodramatic) symbolic content of those messages, play a key role in 'the social amplification and attenuation of risk' (Kasperson and Kasperson 1996).

In this regard, it is perhaps interesting to note that, back on 3 September 1966, Jerome D. Frank used his presidential address to the Society for the Psychological Study of Social Issues to ask why technological risks to our environment, particularly in relation to the hazards of nuclear energy, appeared to weigh so little in the minds of the American public (Frank 1966: 1–14). At that time, what seemed most remarkable to Frank was the extent to which the hazards of radioactivity and chemical toxins remained outside the sphere of public debate. In this context, 'risk consciousness' was debatable largely in terms of its absence, and he was inclined to view the public's complacency on these issues as an inevitable consequence of the extent to which they were liable to be preoccupied with more perceptibly immediate material concerns. Nevertheless, writing when television had only recently been established in the majority of households as an affordable mass medium of news and entertainment, he identified 'grounds for hope' in the potential for it to be used 'to speed the changes in public attitudes required by the changes in the environment' (ibid.: 13).

I wonder what Frank would make of the contrasts between our present cultural reality as compared to that of thirty-five years ago? There is now a huge industry of social and psychological research committed to analysing the ways in which 'the public' appear to be morbidly preoccupied with technological risks to their health and the natural environment, indeed, a number of specialist journals are devoted to the study of this topic. Moreover, in this context researchers are certainly unlikely to consider the mass media to be lacking any enthusiasm when it comes to the coverage of technological and environmental hazards. Indeed, in recent years, where governments and large corporations have made massive investments into the practice of 'risk management' (Adams 1995: 31–2), within the field of 'risk communication' one is likely to find the content of news media messages being blamed for fanning the flames of 'moral panic' in relation to technological risk (Graham and Wiener 1995: 6; Kasperson and Kasperson 1996; Leiss 1996; Powell and Leiss 1997). Matters of risk now appear as a grave 'public concern', and there are many who hold the mass media largely responsible for cultivating a fundamental transformation in our perspectives on nature and society.

Accordingly, I would place a heavy emphasis upon the extent to which the task of interpreting the significance of risk consciousness for anxiety is inextricably bound up with debates surrounding the impact of modern forms of communication media upon our cultural experience of modernity. When it comes to evaluating contrasting perspectives on the risk–anxiety relationship, then to a large extent this will be heavily influenced by our understanding of the ways in which the content of media messages *effect* and/or *reflect* the thoughts and feelings of their audiences. Where we venture to comment upon 'the risk debate' in social science, then we cannot leave aside the question of the extent to which our knowledge and experience of the world are shaped according to the logic of 'mediated' symbolic representations of reality which are unique to the dynamics of a society constituted by systems of mass communication (Murdoch 1993; Thompson 1995).

In what follows, I will attempt to outline some contrasting conceptions of the relationship between the media, risk and anxiety. Moreover, in continuing a dominant theme of previous chapters, I will consider the conflict of interpretations which characterises debates in this area as ultimately instructive for the ways in which we evaluate the significance of 'risk consciousness' for anxiety. Furthermore, in this context, I am inclined to emphasise the extent to which attempts at settling matters on the basis of empirical research may be considered as having the overall effect of exposing the inadequacy of our theoretical concepts for dealing with the complexity of this issue. The more empirical information we gather on the ways in which people *actively* interpret and negotiate with the meanings of media messages, the harder it is to reach any definitive conclusions about the impact of those messages upon a population's thoughts and feelings. Accordingly, where some would persuade us towards a definitive point of view on the risk–anxiety relationship, I would highlight the extent to which this requires us to adopt the simplifying logic of abstract speculations which may do no more than leave us building castles in the air.

## The question of content

If any doubts are to be cast on the reality of 'risk consciousness', then you can be sure that there is no shortage of commentators who would direct us to the content of news media as clear evidence to the contrary (Massumi 1993; Furedi 1997). On any single day our newspapers are filled with accounts of violent crime, war, disease, environmental hazards, toxins in our food and people coming to harm as a consequence of the failings of health and scientific experts. Moreover, in television news we have a daily catalogue of hazard, which more often than not, is brought to our attention with the aid of some of the most 'spectacular' imagery of disaster that modern technology can produce. It is with dramatic scenes of the most horrific consequences of an airplane crash that the risks of air travel are brought to public concern; it is with representations of terrible injury and violence that we are most likely to be alerted to the risk of becoming the victim of crime; and more often than not, it is with the most tragic accounts of personal affliction that we are alerted to risks to our health. On this evidence, 'risk consciousness' may be identified not so much in terms of a rounded debate on the 'reality' of possible future hazards, but rather, with reference to the imagery of disaster and personal tragedy. Indeed, as far as Eleanor Singer and Phyllis Endreny are concerned, 'media do not report risks, they report harms' (Singer and Endreny 1987: 10). Similarly, Lee Wilkins and Philip Patterson emphasise that, 'news does not report risk but rather the negative consequences of assuming that risk' (Wilkins and Patterson 1987: 82).

It is in reaction to this fact that in the context of risk management considerable efforts are being made to direct the terms of public debate on risk away from languages of death and destruction, towards a more inclusive representation of expert assessments of the costs and benefits of industrial technologies and scientific experiments. For example, in the analysis of writers such as Douglas Powell and William Leiss, effective risk communication essentially concerns the task of bringing 'scientific' opinion to bear upon the terms of public debate so as to balance public concerns about coming to harm with a message about the 'reality' of danger from the perspective of expert analysis. On this view, it is hoped that 'the public' might ultimately be persuaded to place a greater amount of trust in the capacity of science to reveal 'the truth' about the 'reality' of risk so as to regard discrete events of tragedy in light of the probability that the vast majority of people can be guaranteed a life of comfort and safety (Powell and Leiss 1997: 26–40).

In this regard, Powell and Leiss are not unusual in holding to the presumption that by analysing the content of media messages they are gaining insights into what is most likely to be going on inside the minds and within the emotions of members of the general public. Indeed, few would dispute that, at the very least, the contents of news media messages are liable to 'keynote' our attempts at making sense of the world of risk 'by helping to structure the lines along which initial discussions proceed' (Stallings 1990: 81). However, among those writers who would persuade us that people are anxiously preoccupied with the remote threat of danger, it is often the case that we find the contents of news media messages being referred to as though they were a *direct* reflection of the thoughts which govern the audience's feelings. On this view, melodramatic reports of disaster, injury and destruction are understood to grip people's imaginations to the extent to which they may well be identified not only as evidence of 'what the public thinks' about particular types of risk, but also, as representative of dominant attitudes towards society.

For example, as we might expect, Ulrich Beck's analysis draws heavily upon the suggestion that where large numbers of people meet each day on the 'village green of television' to watch the evening news, then their 'susceptibility to crises' grows (Beck 1992: 132–3; 1995: 100). Moreover, as far as Brian Massumi is concerned, fearful news media reports on death, destruction and personal tragedy not only reflect the popular view that 'a general disaster is already upon us, woven into the fabric of day-to-day life' (Massumi 1993: 11), but further, he identifies a key role for the mass media in cultivating this pervasive sense of panic. Accordingly, Massumi goes so far as to suggest that, 'the media affect – fear-blur – is the direct collective perception of the contemporary condition of the possibility of being human' (ibid.: 24). Similarly, it is with an almost exclusive focus upon the contents of news media 'scare stories' about risks to our health and threats to our children that Frank Furedi would convince us that contemporary society is now held in thrall to the 'culture of fear' (Furedi 1997).

By contrast, I am inclined to emphasise that, in light of the increasing amounts of empirical data that are gathered on the ways in which people perceive the risks they face, and in particular where this is considered in relation to qualitative studies of the social contexts in which audiences *actively* interpret the meanings of media messages, then it becomes extremely difficult to determine the cultural significance of such mediated forms of 'risk consciousness'. Indeed, what becomes more remarkable is the extent to which the processes of discourse through which people may occasionally negotiate the meaning of their world in terms of risk, appear to be comprised of a range of partial opinions, ambiguous responses and contradictory views about public sphere debates on the social problems of our times. Moreover, in this regard considerable doubts may be cast upon the presumption that large numbers of people are becoming anxiously preoccupied by the information they receive on risk via the medium of 'news'; in fact, what may be more noteworthy is the extent to which, while having an 'awareness' of these issues, people appear to spend little time actually worrying about the possibilities of being personally 'at risk'. However, perhaps above all else, what becomes most apparent is the inadequacy of our conceptual frameworks for accounting for the complexity of social processes of symbolic production and exchange

## The quality of risk perception

In recent years, perceived risk has become a major interest of policy-makers, political commentators and sociological researchers. However, there is still no consensus when it comes to determining the precise meaning of 'risk perception' and certainly, there is no agreement as to how one should interpret the data of empirical studies designed to reveal how people make interpretations of 'hazard' as 'risk' (Coleman 1993: 612–13; Cutter 1993: 11–32; Sjoberg 1997; 1998; 2000; Brenot *et al.* 1998; Irwin *et al.* 1999). Indeed, with this in mind, it may be surprising to note that, despite the expansive literature on this subject in the domain of academe, there are no clear empirical grounds for accepting that society is now more 'risk conscious' than it has ever been in the past. Indeed, it is not only the case that there is still no agreement as to how people think and feel about the risks they face, but also, the very existence of 'risk consciousness' as a dominant mentality of Western societies remains open to debate. It may well be the case that this is in no small part due to the conflicting range of interpretations which characterise attempts at understanding the interrelationship between members of society and news media representations of risk.

Nevertheless, it is certainly the case that in looking at the evidence of opinion polls one might well conclude that the populations of Western societies are increasingly preoccupied with matters of risk. For example, in the past twenty years it appears that there is a heightening awareness of risks to the environment (Anthony 1982; Dunlap and Scarce 1991; ONS 1998: 187–90; Young 1990). Indeed, according to the European Commission's 1995 *Eurobarometer Survey*, a clear majority of the populations of the member states of the European Union now consider the task of 'protecting the environment and fighting pollution' to be 'an immediate and urgent problem' (ONS 1998: 188). Moreover, it appears that it is particularly in relation to the hazards of nuclear, chemical and industrial technologies that people are inclined to perceive the greatest amounts of risk to nature and society (Young 1990; ONS 1998: 188). On these findings, it would seem that a writer such as Ulrich Beck is fully justified in identifying 'risk consciousness' as a major preoccupation of our times.

Furthermore, one might present a strong case for considering this new consciousness of environmental risk as a direct result of the influence of mass media (Young 1990: 78). For example, William Gamson and André Modigliani (1989) suggest that the 'interpretive packages' which were used by Western news media to report the catastrophes at Three Mile Island and Chernobyl have had a major structuring effect upon the American population's attitudes towards the risks of nuclear technology. Accordingly, where opinion polls may be used to chart the growth of public hostility towards the nuclear industry, they note that this seems to develop in correspondence with the appearance of a more strident anti-nuclear power discourse in Western news media. Similarly, Allan Mazur maintains that there is a direct link between the findings of opinion poll surveys on support for new scientific/technological developments and the amount of media coverage of accidents and hazards. Indeed, in this regard he argues that:

> [T]he quantity of coverage of a technical controversy can have as much effect on public attitudes as the semantic content of the stories that are presented. The public takes seriously any suggestion that a technology may be risky, particularly if the suggestion is repeated often enough. Whilst this shows a discriminating public that does not blithely embrace every new scientific innovation that is wrapped in a pretty package, it also shows a public with anxieties.
>
> (Mazur 1981: 14)

By contrast, there are a number of writers who cast suspicion on this view. For example, Anders Hansen argues that we should not understand opinion polls to provide us with much of an insight into the issues which members of society worry about in the contexts of everyday life but, rather, it is more appropriate to consider them to be charting the public's awareness of what mass media identify for them as topics of social concern (Hansen 1991: 444–5). Accordingly, the findings of attitudinal surveys may bear little or no connection to matters of personal anxiety, but rather be simply documenting our general knowledge of the symbolic representation of society's problems in the public sphere. Indeed, such an interpretation is likely to find support among researchers investigating the 'impersonal impact hypothesis', which suggests that people are inclined to separate what they perceive as risks to society from what they understand as risks to themselves (Coleman 1993; Culbertson and Stempel 1985; Tyler and Cook 1984). On this view, we might well anticipate that, in light of melodramatic news media reports on the major hazards of our times, people will perceive there to be a 'crime problem', 'health risk' or 'ecological crisis' *for society*, however, when asked about the extent to which they consider themselves to be *personally* 'at risk' from these dangers, we should expect them to be far more optimistic about their prospects for living in safety. Thus, one should exercise extreme caution when it comes to using the evidence of opinion polls as a means of establishing how people view risks to society and themselves, for these are not necessarily one and the same thing; while expressing a pessimistic view about risk in society, the majority of people may give little thought to how this relates to their own lives.

It is in recognition of such interpretative dilemmas that a number of writers in the field of risk perception are now inclined to emphasise how little we know about the ways in which people actually perceive the risks they face (Cutter 1993: 10–32; Sjoberg 2000). The more researchers move from simply noting the public's general awareness of public debates about risk towards the problem of determining *how* people perceive the risks they face, as well as the extent to which perception of risk implies worry about risk (Sjoberg 1998), then it appears much harder to reach any definitive conclusions about the social distribution and significance of 'risk consciousness'. Indeed, I am inclined to suggest that it is precisely the inconsistency of research results and the conflicting range of interpretations which are given to data that becomes instructive for building towards a greater understanding of how we might make sense of these issues (Wilkinson 2001).

While it is acknowledged that factors such as gender, age, occupation, geography and ethnicity may all have a significant bearing upon the ways in which people identify and judge the severity of the risks they face, few consistent relationships have been observed between these variables and the social distribution of risk perception (Brenot *et al.* 1998; Cutter 1993: 27–8). Moreover, in light of the discovery that contrasting methodological approaches provide us with quite different and even contradictory accounts of risk perception, then one might suspect that understandings are shaped more as a reflection of research design than in accordance with 'real' insights into the contents of people's thoughts and feelings about these matters. For example, Per Gustafson (1998) argues that current understandings of differences between male and female perceptions of risk are liable to be heavily distorted as a consequence of the majority of risk researchers' preference for using quantitative methodologies (Fischoff *et al.* 1978; 1981;1984; Fife-Schaw and Rowe 1996; Gardner and Gould 1989; Slovic 1987). He argues that where the measurements of the dominant psychometric paradigm in risk perception research use comparisons between the results of questionnaires which work according to the assumption that men and women worry about similar types of issues and use the same criteria of interpretation for giving meanings to the problems they face, then they may fail to recognise some of the most important *qualities* of difference between the ways we perceive risk (Gustafson 1998: 806). In this regard, Gustafson notes that more qualitative approaches reveal men and women not only perceive the same risks in different ways but also worry about different types of risk (Cutter *et al.* 1992). Accordingly, where researchers present us with orders of perceived risk and measurements of 'dread', these are suspected on the grounds that the full range of respondents' attitudes and perceptions are severely under-represented, or even largely absent, from the results of questionnaires with closed options of reply; the meanings which people give to the risks they face may well be far more subtle and varied than is presumed by research design.

Indeed, in the rarer instances where researchers use qualitative methodologies to inquire into the ways in which people use the language of risk and negotiate with its meaning within the social contexts of everyday life, then it appears that the reality of risk perception is considerably more complex and ambiguous than current terms of analysis might suggest (Bellaby 1990; Irwin *et al.* 1999). A good example of this is to be found in a study conducted by Alan Irwin and colleagues into the ways in which members of the community of Jarrow reason about industrial hazards as a risk to their local environment. In this context, it is evidently the case that people hold to few fixed perspectives on risk, rather, their understandings are immersed within a dialogical process where at any one time an individual may hold to a range of partial and inconsistent views. These writers emphasise the importance of social context for understanding the ways in which people negotiate the meaning of risk; during the course of a single day an individual may express a range of contrasting opinions about the risks they face depending upon the company they keep and the social activities they are engaged in. Accordingly, they argue that lay understandings of risk are fundamentally 'heterogeneous in character' and conclude that:

> [A]n important characteristic of lay understandings and responses . . . is that they do not exist in some neatly packaged form for researchers to collect and take away. Instead of serving as knowledge repositories, local people actively create forms of understanding as they negotiate the conditions of everyday life. This also suggests the resourceful and creative manner in which new situations and issues can be dealt with: various sources and types of evidence are brought together (including personal experience, human and nonhuman evidence, local memories), moral and personal judgements are expressed, those with particular expertise or experience are consulted (and, periodically, challenged), arguments are tested out and modified.
>
> (Irwin *et al.* 1999: 1322)

Moreover, in the context of media research this emphasis upon the ways in which individuals are actively involved in the social process of producing a diversity of meanings for topics of public debate may now be identified as among the most well-supported conclusions of contemporary audience studies. Indeed, where ethnographic research reveals that individuals in the act of interpreting the content of media messages, may construct a great variety of meanings out of what they see, hear and read which are quite different to those of experts in media analysis, then commentators have become far more reluctant to reach any definitive conclusions about the power of mass media to 'affect' our thoughts, feelings and behaviour (Ang 1991; Kitzinger 1999; Lull 1990;1991; McLeod *et al.* 1991; Morley 1986; 1992; Morley and Silverstone 1990; Silverstone 1994). Accordingly, as audience researchers have become increasingly sensitive towards the importance of social context for understanding the ways in which people make sense of the terms of public debate and incorporate its significance into their everyday conversations and activities (Dahlgren 1988), then we may be sure that Roger Silverstone represents a widely shared point of view when declaring that a 'considerable indeterminacy [lies] at the heart of our understanding of the audience' (Silverstone 1994: 143).

Some of the recent work conducted by members of the Glasgow Media Group may be used to illustrate the importance of this view for conceptualising the interrelationship between news media messages and 'risk consciousness'. In examining audience reactions to a variety of contemporary risk issues such as AIDS, BSE ('mad cow disease'), child sexual abuse and terrorism, they maintain that there is most certainly no homogeneous type of audience response to the content of news media messages on these problems. Their qualitative research reveals that people read a great variety of meanings into the content of news and that this appears to be influenced not only by differences in the 'quality' of information received but also according to the peculiarity of individual social circumstances. Jenny Kitzinger comments:

> Diversity was not only related to differences in media consumption, conflicting information between different media outlets and reader 'selectivity'. It also related to people's social, political and personal positions and identifications. People used their identities, knowledge and politics around class, racism and gender relations to engage critically with media representations across all the topics we examined.
>
> (Kitzinger 1999: 13)

Among other things, it is due to their recognition of such factors that I consider the work of David Miller and Jacqui Reilly on 'food scares' to provide us with one of the best examples of how we might begin to map out the complexity of the processes of communication involved in the (possible) development of forms of 'risk consciousness' among the general public (Miller and Reilly 1994; Reilly 1999). In the first instance, they emphasise that where an issue such as 'salmonella in eggs' becomes a topic of 'news', this most certainly should *not* be considered as a direct reflection of levels of public concern surrounding the risks of eating eggs, but rather, it is more likely to appear as a result of the political power of news sources such as the National Farmers Union, the Department of Health and the Ministry of Agriculture to dictate the terms of public debate on behalf of their own minority concerns. Accordingly, it appears that the length of time that 'salmonella in eggs' remained as an issue on the public agenda bore no immediate relationship to the amounts of anxiety experienced and/or expressed by members of 'the public', but rather, was most clearly a consequence of the failure of these organisations to decide among themselves on the correct definition of this 'problem' in the arena of public debate (Hilgartner and Bosk 1988). On this view, 'salmonella in eggs' only remained in the news so long as these organisations conceived their economic and political interests to lie in directing the terms of public debate towards their favoured rendition of the alleged 'problem'; once the National Farmers Union was recognised by the others as having won the battle for definition, then this issue disappeared from the news media agenda (Miller and Reilly 1994). Indeed, even when the risk of contracting salmonella from eggs was technically assessed as greater in the mid-1990s than it was during the 'egg scare' of winter 1988 (Eldridge 1999: 120–5), now that these particular news sources have agreed upon the terms of risk discourse on eggs, then this issue hardly ever appears as a topic of public concern.

It is more specifically in relation to 'the BSE crisis' that Jacqui Reilly has made an attempt at identifying some of the ways in which people may think and feel in response to these debates. Once again what becomes clear is the extent to which public perceptions of risk are never fixed or constant but, rather, subject to the dynamics of cultural *processes* in which people are liable to be actively involved in creating and holding to a range of contrasting points of view. The results of her in-depth interviews conducted over a four-year period reveal a highly complex process of interaction between news media and their audiences. In this example, what is most striking is not only people's ability to refer to a wide variety of sources of influence when talking about BSE, but also the extent to which opinions are open to be modified both in response to new information and in reflection upon other lifestyle variables. It is evidently the case that the cultural significance of this particular 'food scare' cannot be considered purely on its own terms; rather, people's opinions are shaped by their responses to other topics of public debate and patterns of media consumption. Moreover, this study reveals that individual attitudes and behaviours may vary considerably over time, not only in relation to changes in the items of news media discourse, but also in response to the general experience of work and family life. In this regard, where people may initially appear to react with a short-term response of anxiety towards a news media report on the risk of contracting BSE, in the long term, due to the wide variety of other daily pressures and life interests which clamour for our attention, the dangers of eating beef may rarely, if at all, be encountered as a major issue for concern.

Such findings are sure to guarantee there will certainly be no consensus when it comes to reaching any decisions upon the extent to which it is appropriate to identify individuals and groups in society as 'risk conscious'. While it is undoubtedly the case that there is a general awareness among members of 'the public' of risk-related issues, there is no agreement among researchers as to how this impacts upon their general attitudes, feelings and behaviours. Indeed, more qualitative approaches suggest that in this regard individuals should not be considered to hold steadfastly to one type of opinion about risk or be inclined towards any single kind of response in relation to the information they receive on threats to their health and the environment. On the one hand, it appears that in the social contexts of 'everyday life' people are certainly subject to the 'influence' of the content of media messages, but on the other, when it comes to determining precisely what this amounts to for individual thoughts and actions, then it appears that we are dealing with forms of cultural complexity which remain poorly accounted for within existing frameworks for theorising the relationship between news media and their audiences. Moreover, it is particularly in light of the ethnographic 'discovery' of the multiple forms of audience 'activity' which impinge upon the ways in which they interpret and respond to the meanings of media messages that I would argue that those seeking to determine the significance of this for our cultural experience of modernity may only consider themselves to be in a position to advance understanding when every effort is made to heed 'the limits of our claims and the incommensurabilities between them' (Silverstone 1994: 133).

## Speculation reigns

Insofar as it appears that there is no definitive account of the cultural processes in which people actively negotiate the meaning of 'risk', then we may be sure that all who would venture to link 'risk consciousness' to the experience of anxiety will at some point be entering into the realms of speculation. As we have seen, there is not only considerable dispute with regard to what constitutes authentic evidence of 'risk consciousness' in society, but also, even where commentators achieve some consensus upon the criteria for gathering reliable data on the social reality of risk perception, the significance of this for the experience of anxiety seems always to remain open to debate. Moreover, where the mass media may be understood to be heavily implicated within the development of forms of cultural experience which dispose us to 'see' the world in terms of risk, we may be sure that there will be no final agreement upon the dynamics of the interrelationship between media, risk and anxiety. There is a persistent conflict of interpretations with regard to the social meanings of the contents of media messages, the cultural significance of risk perception, as well as the quality of people's everyday worries and concerns.

We may anticipate that within the complexity of the social dynamics of communication flows, that which one writer sees as signs of anxiety another will consider as clear evidence to the contrary. For example, Roger Silverstone argues that where certain items in the content of news may certainly be viewed as a potential source of anxiety, there is much in the presentational style and format of television news programmes which is just as likely to reassure audiences that all is well in the world. He argues:

> the levels of anxiety that could be raised (and of course may well be either inevitably or deliberately raised) are ameliorated both in terms of the structure of the news as a programme (the tidying of papers, mutual smiles and silent chat following a 'human interest' story complete news over the world), and in terms of its reliability and frequency.
>
> (Silverstone 1994: 16–17)

Similarly, Patricia Mellencamp (1990) emphasises the possibility that where at one moment the flow of news may be experienced as a source of anxiety, in the next, it has the potential to become a form of therapy. With particular reference to television news coverage of a national catastrophe she suggests that when a 'news flash' suddenly interrupts the regular sequence of programming to announce the event of disaster, then in the first instance, this may well be encountered as a source of anxiety. However, with constant up-to-the-minute news coverage, the in-depth analysis of causes and consequences as well as the rational calm of the broadcaster's presentational styles, then audiences are also likely to use television as a means of coping with the trauma of their experience. Working with reference to Freud's later writings on the problem of anxiety (Freud 1979), she argues that in this context, television may be understood to be heavily involved with the orchestration of a cultural process where it is possible to interpret the contents of media messages as both the cause of anxiety and as an aid to emotional catharsis. On this analysis, it is suggested that when at one point in time the melodramatic contents of the first news of disaster may make people vulnerable to experience the 'indefiniteness' of anxiety, nevertheless *with* time, the drive to supply an 'objective' meaning for the events in question is most likely to provide viewers with a means of diffusing their momentary feelings of helplessness so as to return to a state of ordered calm. For Mellencamp, one of the most memorable early examples of television's dual capacity for 'shock and therapy' was made apparent in the immediate aftermath of the assassination of John F. Kennedy. After the initial period of social alarm, she maintains that television news was used to build a sense of 'collective identification' whereby 'the populace [was] united, soothed, and finally ennobled by repetition of and patient waiting for information' (Mellencamp 1990: 254).

Accordingly, when seeking to account for the dynamics of the interrelationship between media, risk and anxiety, we should be alert to the fact that we are dealing with cultural processes where from one minute to the next people may move through a range of different thoughts and feelings. In this regard, it may be entirely inappropriate to consider this to offer us any vantage point for revealing the presiding cultural character of our current period of modernity. To generalise upon the meaning of the anxiety of our times on the basis of any single 'snapshot' account of how people appeared and/or reported themselves to be thinking and feeling about any particular risk is always liable to court controversy, for in this process it seems that at different times and places there may be much more (or indeed much less) to the world than any single evaluation of our cultural situation would suggest is the case.

While as a matter of speculation, it remains possible that in the long term, the cumulative 'effect' of news media coverage of different types of health and environmental hazards may cultivate 'a generalised climate of risk' (Giddens 1991: 109) or a pervasive sense of anxiety about the 'dangerousness' of the world (Bryant et al. 1981: 106–11), within the social dynamics of our interactions with 'mediated' information on risk there are many other interpretations which may be given to the ways in which this is liable to 'influence' our thoughts, feelings and behaviours. Moreover, where in this context it appears that empirical research may be used in support of a range of contrasting points of view, then, at some point, all accounts of the interrelationship between media, risk and anxiety may be identified more as an artefact of research design than as a genuine advance towards discovering the 'facts' about our common experience of society (Wober and Gunter 1982).

It may well be the case that by emphasising the inadequacy of our methodological and theoretical frameworks for dealing with the complexity of the cultural dynamics through which people negotiate the meaning of the world in terms of risk, then we may move closer to revealing something of 'the truth' about the interrelationship between 'risk consciousness' and the experience of anxiety. Indeed, in this matter I am inclined to endorse David Byrne's contention that 'the point about complexity is that it is useful – it helps us to understand the things we are trying to understand' (Byrne 1998: 7). Accordingly, when inquiring into the character of 'risk consciousness', what may be most important to recognise is the extent to which it is precisely in relation to an experience of cultural complexity which resists categorisation within the static abstractions of conceptual analysis that people may be moved to adopt the language of risk for explaining and expressing their anxieties (Irwin et al. 1999; Wilkinson 2001).

However, in the final analysis I am inclined towards the view that it may be largely due to the problem of anxiety itself that it is only within the context of theoretical speculation that we may venture to determine the cultural significance of 'risk consciousness' in our times. Where up to this point, as a means of emphasising the inevitable conflicting interpretations which may be given to the risk–anxiety relationship, I have sought to highlight something of the complexity of the socially experienced meanings of our mediated cultural reality, above all else, it is with particular reference to the peculiarity of the phenomenological or existential meaning of anxiety that I would emphasise that speculation reigns in any attempt at determining the ways in which public debates on risk 'reflect' or 'effect' current thoughts and feelings about the world in which we find ourselves.

## The problem of anxiety for a risk society

One of my principal aims in writing this book is to draw the problem of anxiety into the purview of the sociological imagination of our times. Where sociologists venture to pass comment upon the relationship between risk consciousness and anxiety, for the most part, this is understood predominantly to concern debates over the meaning of 'risk' and the cultural/political significance of 'risk debate' in the public sphere; the problem of anxiety, considered on its own terms, is generally not recognised to be in need of any substantive sociological analysis. However, from the outset of my discussion I have worked according to the critical suggestion that where the risk–anxiety relationship is open to a range of conflicting interpretations, then this may be identified not only as a consequence of sociological disputes over the cultural significance of 'risk consciousness', but also as a result of the complexity of the problems which anxiety brings to our lives. Indeed, where in previous chapters attempts have been made to explore some of these problems in sociological perspective, as a presiding theme of inquiry I have sought to emphasise that, so long as we are specifically concerned to advance an understanding of anxiety, then we should anticipate that there will be no final agreement upon the proper meaning of this condition, let alone its precise causes and prevalence in modern societies.

Of course, as an elemental point of analysis, insofar as anxiety may be identified as a cultural experience which is common to us all, then we should expect people to acquire and create many different meanings for the problems it brings to their lives. Moreover, in this regard alone we may anticipate that even where concerted attempts are made to put theories to the test in the domain of empirical research, then there will be no consensus when it comes to the right way of interpreting the results. As Max Weber comments:

> One thing is certain under all circumstances, namely, the more 'general' the problem involved, i.e. in this case, the broader its cultural *significance* (*sic*), the less subject it is to a single unambiguous answer on the basis of empirical sciences and the greater the role played by value-ideas (*Wertideen*) and the ultimate and highest axioms of belief.
>
> (Weber 1949: 56 – emphasis in original)

However, in addition to this, I have raised the critical suggestion that where the negative quality of the experience of anxiety appears to take place in the context of personal encounters with situations of foreboding obscurity, then this also may be identified as a contributing factor to ongoing disputes over the 'reality' of this condition. I would have us consider the extent to which it may be due to the peculiarity of the phenomena of anxiety that we should not be surprised to discover that 'there are as many conceptions of anxiety as there are theories of man' (Fischer 1970: 135).

Following authorities such as Freud and Kierkegaard, I have consistently sought to refer the reader to the extent to which the experience of anxiety (in contradistinction to fear) has a 'quality of indefiniteness' (Freud 1979: 325) which always leaves people searching for symbolic forms of culture which are adequate to the task of expressing its 'true' origins and identity. On this view, where people remain caught in the grip of anxiety, then we should expect them to be left feeling frustrated in the knowledge that our culture has yet to provide them with a sufficient means of overcoming, or avoiding the sense of being overwhelmed by the threatening uncertainty of future possibilities. Accordingly, I have argued that where there is always uncertainty in the lived experience of anxiety, then this itself may be sufficient to ensure that the precise causes and constituent aspects of this condition remain open to debate.

I suggest that we are dealing with a form of experience which is fundamentally constituted by our capacity for speculation. In its most distressing forms, anxiety appears to be borne by consciousness as a problem of meaning which so aggravates us that we are driven to engage in a speculative search for the 'truth' about the feeling that something is seriously wrong with our world.

Indeed, so long as it may be basic to our humanity that we are prone to anxiety, then I suspect that we shall always be inclined towards the conviction that there is a deficit of meaning in the world. Thus, in the final analysis, I would argue that so long as we are specifically concerned to account for the problem of anxiety in contemporary societies, then we should expect that doubts will continue to cast their shadow over any favoured representation of the cultural reality of this condition in our times. Where anxiety makes itself known to all, its 'real' identity is always kept obscure; thus, its cultural significance will remain open to interpretation.

For these reasons I suspect that there will always be work for the 'sociological imagination' in identifying public issues to bring a greater 'objectivity' to bear upon people's experiences of anxiety so that they might have an explicit focus for their fears (Mills 1959: 3–24). Accordingly, where C. Wright Mills would have us identify the value of sociology in its 'promise' to perform the cultural task of overcoming the uneasy suspense of anxiety by exposing the political significance of the relationship between public issues of structure to the personal troubles of milieu, I consider him to present us with an unlimited project. If people may be convinced that it is by cultivating more of a 'sociological imagination' that they may begin to feel more 'at home' in the world, then we may anticipate that this discipline will always have justification to keep itself at work.

On this view, I consider Zygmunt Bauman to provide us with a fitting epitaph for the cultural history of our humanity when he comments:

> Each era of history had its own fears which set it apart from other epochs; or rather, each gave the fears known to all epochs names of its own creation. These names were concealed interpretations; they informed of where the roots of the feared threats lay, what one could do to keep the threats away, or why one could do nothing to ward them off.
>
> (Bauman 1995: 105)

As with fear, so with anxiety. Indeed, in modern times it is with particular regard to those fears whose roots remain obscure and which we conceive to present us with no clear means of escape that we have come to explicitly refer to 'the sting of fear' in terms of the problem of anxiety (Tillich 1952: 46; May 1977: 3–19). It is in this context that I would have us identify languages of risk as just one of the many ways in which people may come to experience, or move to appease, the tension between our knowledge and ignorance of fearful situations. In the cultural history of anxiety, I would present narratives on risk as a further attempt, which follows in the wake of many more besides, to bring the work of reason to bear upon the uneasiness of anxiety so as to make up the deficit of meaning whereby this condition leaves us in the distress of feeling that something is fearfully wrong with our world. Moreover, I suspect that so long as anxiety remains, there will be many more stories for us to write about ourselves; there will always be a need for new concepts to bestow meaning upon the anxieties of our human condition. Indeed, perhaps it is the fate of all attempts to give meaning to anxiety that they end at the point of exhaustion?

For now, we may still be in the process of discovering the possible ways in which the concept of risk may be used as a means of making sense of our anxieties. It is only recently that a number of books have appeared on the market which, while establishing the concept of risk as one of the unit ideas (Nisbet 1966: 5–6) of contemporary sociology, make an attempt at locating groups of writers within distinct sub-disciplines and theoretical schools (Lupton 1999a; 1999b; Adam *et al.* 2000). As with any concept which gains such wide appeal, its proper definition cannot be made subject to the rule of any individual authority or tradition of sociological inquiry. Within the sociology of risk there is certainly no theoretical consensus as to the 'objective' reality of the risks we face, likewise, when it comes to the cultural meaning of 'risk consciousness' we are faced with a conflict of interpretations. Indeed, much debate still surrounds the question of whether this is even an appropriate term for describing the dominant mentality of our times.

For my part, I find myself with most sympathy towards writers who place the greater emphasis upon the extent to which the experienced reality of risk is a social construct which is brought into being by 'a heterogeneous network of interactive actors, institutions, knowledges and practices' (Lupton 1999a: 87). On this view, the sociological task is to identify the specific social conditions in which people come to know and interact with 'risk' as a product of particular power discourses or techniques of rationalisation for bestowing a meaningful order upon reality (Dean 1999; Crook 1999; Culpitt 1999; O'Malley 1996). Accordingly, I am inclined to endorse Mitchell Dean's contention that:

> the [sociological] significance of risk does not lie with risk itself but with what risk gets attached to . . . What is important about risk is not risk itself, but the forms of knowledge that make it thinkable from statistics, sociology and epidemiology to management and

accounting, the techniques that discover it from the calculus of probabilities to the interview, the social technologies that seek to govern
it from risk screening, case-management and social insurance to situational crime prevention, and the political rationalities and
programmes that deploy it, from those that dreamt of a welfare state
to those that imagine an advanced liberal society of prudential individuals and communities.

(Dean 1999: 131–2)

In this regard there is a pressing need to make theoretical discussions more subject to the critical force of empirical studies exploring the ways in which people
experience and use knowledge about risk in the contexts of their everyday lives.
Certainly, where efforts are made in this direction, there appears to be good
cause to suspect the abstractions of grand theory for presenting us with notions
of social reality which seriously underestimate the heterogeneous character of
risk language and debate under conditions of 'everyday life' (Irwin *et al.* 1999).
Where sociological risk discourse takes place largely within the context of a theoretical debate on the character of modernity, much work remains to be done in
bringing this to a proper recognition of the social and cultural complexity of the
'risk society' as it is experienced and made by people in their particular
localities.

In this book I have begun to explore some of the ways in which the concept
of risk may be 'attached to' sociological debates on the problem of anxiety in
modern societies. I have sought to identify some contrasting conceptions of
the risk–anxiety relationship, and further, I have attempted to explain these not
only in relation to the semantics of risk, but also in connection with the peculiarity of the condition of anxiety itself. Indeed, as a point of emphasis, I
would urge the reader to consider the extent to which, in the final analysis, it
may be due to the complexity of the problem of meaning in anxiety that we
should anticipate that there will always be many different ways of interpreting the contents of our experience according to the semantics of risk.
However, where my analysis has been conducted largely as a matter of theoretical debate, I consider there to be a great need for further work to expose
the empirical reality of the risk–anxiety relationship. Moreover, in this regard,
what may be most interesting to discover is not only the specific ways in
which people may be moved to conceive their everyday experience of anxiety
in terms of the language of risk, but also the political contexts in which risk
discourse may be used as a conduit for associating affairs of public debate
with our everyday experience of anxiety.

## Conclusion

Over the last two chapters I have focused my discussion more directly upon the contention that society is more anxious because it is more risk conscious. I have outlined a range of contrasting starting points for embarking upon a critical analysis of the risk–anxiety relationship. I have consistently sought to refer the reader to the extent to which the meaning of this relationship is held subject to a conflict of interpretations. Indeed, I would have us consider the extent to which it is by recognising that there are no final certainties with regard to the meaning of 'risk consciousness' for anxiety (or vice versa), that we may be in a better position to assess the cultural and political significance of these particular ways of thinking and feeling about our world.

In the previous chapter this point was explored more directly in relation to the hermeneutics of risk. Here I have dwelled in more analytical detail upon Ulrich Beck's contention that 'the risk society marks the dawning of a speculative age in everyday perception and thought' (Beck 1992: 73). To a large extent this has been explored in relation to the task of conceptualising and evaluating the cultural significance of the interrelationship between media, risk and anxiety. However, in the final analysis I have focused particular attention upon the extent to which the problem of anxiety itself is liable to ensure that, where we venture to account for the experienced reality of a 'risk society' we shall always be entering into the realms of speculation. In these contexts, I have sought to expose some of the theoretical and political commitments which appear to have a determining effect upon contrasting sociological accounts of the cultural significance of risk for the experience of anxiety. Furthermore, I have been concerned to highlight the inadequacies of our theoretical and methodological frameworks for handling the social and cultural complexities of the risk–anxiety relationship, particularly insofar as this comes under the 'influence' of mediated processes of symbolic production and exchange. However, above all else, I have been working with the aim of making the problem of anxiety itself a matter for sociological investigation. I would have us consider some of the ways in which this may be used to establish a critical vantage point for making a fuller assessment of the social origins and dimensions of risk consciousness in our times.

# 6

## Conclusion

On reflecting upon the course of intellectual inquiry into the nature of our human condition, Erich Fromm held to the view that:

> Every discovery which has been made and will be made has a long history in which the truth contained in it finds a less and less veiled and distorted expression and approaches more and more adequate formulations. The development of scientific thought is not one in which old statements are discarded as false and replaced by new and correct ones; it is rather a process of continuous reinterpretation of older statements, by which their true kernel is freed from distorting elements . . . the way of scientific progress is constructive reinterpretation of basic visions.
>
> (Fromm 1944: 380)

However, I am inclined towards the view that it is not in every instance that the process of reinterpretation leads to a more complete account of the 'truth' about ourselves. On this point, perhaps Fromm underestimated the potential for the course of scientific discovery to sometimes do more to distort the truths expressed in 'basic visions' than it does to reveal these in their most vital aspects. Indeed, while writing this book I have more often been impressed by the discovery that it is by returning to examine some of the earliest accounts of anxiety as the 'nodal point at which the most important questions [of our humanity] converge' (Freud 1991: 441), that we may be left with a greater appreciation of the elements of distortion which have crept into the ways in which we assess the cultural reality of our times.

Accordingly, where in earlier chapters, an attempt was made at detailing a sociological conception of the problem of anxiety, I am inclined to consider this essentially as a work of hermeneutical recovery; for here I offered no new interpretations of anxiety, rather, I was simply concerned to return to a 'basic vision' of this condition as not so much a matter of personal pathology, but more a sign that something is seriously wrong with the condition of our social world. By referring the reader back to some of the critical issues raised in the (now neglected) works of writers such as Karen Horney and Erich Fromm, I was returning to some elemental points of interpretation for establishing the lines along which my inquiry was to proceed.

By representing anxiety as an expression of the social predicaments and cultural contradictions which comprise our experiences of everyday life, I do not consider myself to have advanced beyond the ground covered by these theorists during the middle decades of the last century. I suggest that a closer reading of their texts may find much more than I have to cast the alleged 'novelty' of our current age of anxiety in critical perspective. Indeed, in terms of their historical sensitivity, the political/ethical principles which guided their terms of inquiry and the intellectual passion with which they set about their task, I consider their insights to have enduring significance for the ways we read meaning into the crisis of our times. Moreover, perhaps the quality of sociological debate is all the more diminished where now this gives no serious consideration to the ideal solutions they envisaged for overcoming the distress of life in modern societies.

For the purposes of this thesis, I was particularly concerned to explore further, and elaborate upon, their understanding of anxiety as a problem of culture; that is, a form of negative experience which is borne by consciousness as a problem of meaning. Above all else, it was by focusing upon the extent to which this might be identified as thriving upon the tension between our knowledge and ignorance of fearful situations, that I sought to establish some critical parameters for analysing the significance of 'risk consciousness' for the experience of anxiety. This was largely a work of theoretical analysis and conceptual debate, and in this context it was necessary to review some of the ways in which the concept of risk now appears as one of the unit ideas of contemporary sociology. However, in the final analysis, I was not so much concerned with what the sociology of risk lends to our understanding of anxiety, but rather, I was working with the aim of developing a critical reading of sociological risk discourse according to the cultural logic(!) of the problem of anxiety. This book was written for the purpose of raising the critical contention that it is by (re)turning the focus of sociological inquiry towards the problem of anxiety itself that we might attain a critical vantage point for exploring the 'reality' of the risk society as it is experienced and made by people in their everyday lives.

To this end, I have repeatedly sought to address the problem of identifying the 'true' origins of our anxieties as well as the task of assessing the overall prevalence of this condition in contemporary societies. I reviewed the empirical evidence to suggest that it is still largely the case that 'love and work' are what matter most for our everyday vulnerability to anxiety. Accordingly, insofar as it may be possible to establish some sociologically 'objective' indicators of the social distribution of anxiety, then the suggestion was made that it is particularly in relation to factors such as the rates of unemployment and divorce that we might begin to piece together the clearest picture of who is likely to be made vulnerable to the most severe (health-threatening) experiences of this condition.

On this analysis, I argued that insofar as it may be possible to establish a link between 'risk consciousness' and the experience of anxiety, we are dealing with cultural processes where the 'reality' of our social situation is far more open to speculation. It is not only the case that much remains to be discovered about the heterogeneous ways in which people perceive risks in the contexts of everyday life, but also, insofar as this involves us in the problem of determining the significance of modern communication media for our cultural experience of modernity, then we are sure to find a range of conflicting interpretations as to the ways in which 'mediated' knowledge about risk 'influences' our understanding of self and society. Accordingly, I sought not only to alert the reader to the extent to which any forthright account of the risk–anxiety relationship is most likely to involve a highly reduced conception of the cultural complexity of this phenomenon, but also to raise the suspicion that where this takes place we may be entering into forms of debate over 'realities' which amount to no more than castles in the air.

This leads me to agree wholeheartedly with Ulrich Beck's contention that if we are to follow his interpretation of our current age of anxiety as a 'risk society', then we must enter into a 'theoretically determined consciousness of reality' (Beck 1992: 73). However, I consider there to be good reason to suspect that there may be aspects to this 'reality' which have no existence beyond the terms of theoretical abstraction. Indeed, where authors such as Ulrich Beck and Mary Douglas appear to be largely unconcerned with the extent to which their theories are either confirmed or denied by the evidence of empirical research, then I raised the critical suggestion that their works are essentially oriented to present us with their favoured political perspectives on the social reality of risk in terms of its ideal representation within theoretical discourses on modernity.

In following this suggestion, when it came to detailing some contrasting sociological conceptions of the risk–anxiety relationship, I began by analysing their significance for opposing theoretical representations of the politics of 'risk consciousness'. I noted that where sociologists venture to comment upon the significance of risk consciousness for the experience of anxiety, in most instances this takes places with the aim of defending a selective point of view on the cultural reality of the risk society; generally speaking, there is no detailed exploration of the problem of anxiety itself outside of a theoretical concern to account for the 'rationality' of this phenomenon as an appropriate response to their judgements upon the magnitude of the risks we face. In this context, I explored how, at the level of conceptual analysis, the semantics of risk may be used to construct opposing hypothetical accounts of the possible causes of anxiety as well as the preferred ways in which people may set about coping with the distress of this condition. However, I was always concerned to emphasise the extent to which there may be a considerable discrepancy between these (politically motivated) ideal constructions of the risk–anxiety relationship and the actual ways in which populations acquire and create knowledge about risk amidst their personal troubles of milieu.

On this basis, when it comes to assessing the cultural significance of risk consciousness for the experience of anxiety, I am inclined towards the view that, for the time being at least, we are largely left with the task of evaluating matters of speculative abstraction. Moreover, where it appears that the sociology of risk is still at the point of discovering the full variety of ways in which this concept may be used to develop existing traditions of inquiry into our cultural experience of modernity, or even to introduce new parameters of debate within the discipline, then it may well be the case that there will be many more accounts for us to consider besides those identified in this book. With this in mind, I aimed not only to explore some of 'the convergences and differences in the insights to risk as a sociocultural phenomenon' (Lupton 1999b: 6), but also, bring the problem of anxiety on its own terms into the purview of the 'sociological imagination' as it seeks to fulfil its promise of interpreting the meaning of 'history and biography and the relationships between the two in society' (Mills 1959: 6).

Where this project gives rise to a conflict of interpretations over the personal and political significance of our current period of cultural history, I have explored this not only in relation to the semantics of risk, but also as a consequence of the phenomenological components of the condition of anxiety itself.

Indeed, insofar as anxiety may be understood to consist in leaving us under the traumatic experience that it is due to our ignorance of the 'reality' of our situation that we are liable to come to harm, then I have suggested that on its own terms, this experience serves as a constant spur to the work of reinterpretation. So long as people are prone to experience anxiety, then we may anticipate that they will always be left feeling that there is more for them to discover about the proper meaning of their human condition. Moreover, in this respect it may be due to the problem of anxiety itself that we should expect there to be no final or definitive account of the risk–anxiety relationship.

In the past sociology may be judged to have fallen short of its 'promise' due to its neglect of the affective dimensions of human existence. With this criticism in mind, I present this narrative as part of the effort to develop a fuller account of our social conditions in terms of the experience of 'inner life'. Much remains to be done in the work of exposing the significance of 'public issues of structure' for the ways we *feel* about the state of our world. Indeed, in this regard, I suspect that we may have only just begun to trace some of the connections between the symbolic forms of culture by which people construct meanings for society and the ways in which these appear to evoke, or are used to express, matters of personal feeling. I hope that I may be judged to have made some progress in clearing the ground for future avenues of inquiry. Moreover, I look forward to the works of those who may yet direct the course of 'constructive reinterpretation' towards greater discoveries of the 'truth' about our experiences of self and society whereby it becomes possible to realise more adequate solutions to the problems which anxiety brings to our lives.

# Notes

## 2  Social indicators of anxiety

1.  As with the concept of anxiety, there are a number of competing definitions of 'stress' (Bartlett 1998: 22–40). Furthermore, researchers are unable to agree upon how we should account for the ways in which the pressures of the external environment interact with our psychology and physiology in order to produce the bodily reaction, which following the pioneering work of Hans Selye (1956; 1974), has come to be referred to as the general adaption syndrome (GAS). The concept of 'stress' is used to refer to 'a particular relationship between the person and the environment that is appraised by the person as taxing or exceeding his or her resources and endangering his or her well-being' (Lazarus and Folkman 1984). Broadly speaking, the experience of stress is conceived in terms of the physical and mental effort it takes to adapt one's lifestyle and behaviour so as to cope with the weight of traumatic life changes and processes of social deprivation. In the majority of studies 'stress' is largely conceived as something which 'happens *to* and *on* the person' (May 1977: 111), rather than an experience connected with the ways in which people acquire and create meanings for their world. For the most part, stress research has remained focused upon the task of explaining the link between bodily stress and ill-health. As far as our biology is concerned, the experience of stress is understood to deteriorate health according to the pressures it places upon the body's immunological, cardiovascular and endocrine systems (Kaplan 1991; Steptoe 1991; Kelly *et al.* 1997; Bartlett 1998: 84–106). The more sociologically oriented approaches are concerned to argue for a causal association between stress and ill-health by focusing upon the extent to which those social groups which are revealed by health statistics as having the highest rates of psychiatric and physical morbidity also tend to experience the most amounts of chronic stressors and negative life events (Pearlin 1989; Elstad 1998).

2. Eric Brunner and Michael Marmot explain:

> Cortisol and other related glucocorticoid hormones have both metabolic and psychological effects. They play a key role in the maintenance and control of resting and stress-related metabolic functions. As antagonists of the hormone insulin, they mobilise energy reserves by raising blood glucose and promoting fatty acid release from fat tissues. During an emergency this is a desirable effect, but in the physically inactive situation the superfluous availability of energy tends to increase output into the blood of cholesterol carrying particles from the liver. The brain is also a target for glucocorticoids, which promote vigilance in the short term. However, a prolonged high level of cortisol . . . can provoke paranoia or depression.
>
> (Brunner and Marmot 1999: 25)

# References

Acheson, D. (1998) *Independent Inquiry into Inequalities in Health: Report*, London: HMSO.

Adam, B., Beck, U. and Van Loon, J. (2000) *The Risk Society and Beyond: Critical Issues for Social Theory*, London: Sage Publications.

Adams, J. (1995) *Risk*, London: UCL Press.

American Psychiatric Association (1994) *Diagnostic and Statistical Manual of Mental Disorders*, 4th edn, Washington, DC: APA.

Anderson, A. (1997) *Media, Culture and the Environment*, London: UCL Press.

Andrews, G. and Peters, L. (1999) *CIDI: The Composite International Diagnostic Interview*, *Discussion Paper*, Geneva: WHO.

Aneshensel, C. (1992) 'Social Stress: Theory and Research', *Annual Review of Sociology* 18: 15–38.

Aneshensel, C., Rutter, C. and Lachenbruch, P. (1991) 'Social Structure, Stress and Mental Health: Competing Conceptual and Analytic Models', *American Sociological Review* 56: 166–78.

Ang, I. (1991) *Desperately Seeking the Audience*, London: Routledge.

Anthony, R. (1982) 'Polls, Pollution and Politics: Trends in Public Opinion on the Environment', *Environment* 24(4): 14–34.

Antonovsky, A. (1979) *Health, Stress and Coping*, San Francisco: Jossey-Bass.

Auden, W. H. (1948) *The Age of Anxiety: A Baroque Eclogue,* London: Faber and Faber.

Ayto, J. (1990) *Dictionary of Word Origins*, London: Columbia Marketing.

Bailey, J. (1988) *Pessimism*, London: Routledge.

Bartlett, D. (1998) *Stress: Perspectives and Processes*, Buckingham: Open University Press.

Bartley, M., Ferrie, J. and Montgomery, S. M. (1999) 'Living in a High-unemployment Economy: Understanding the Health Consequences', in M. Marmot and R. G. Wilkinson (eds) *Social Determinants of Health*, Oxford: Oxford University Press.

Bauman, Z. (1987) *Legislators and Interpreters: On Modernity, Post-Modernity and Intellectuals*, Cambridge: Polity Press.

—— (1992) *Intimations of Postmodernity*, London: Routledge.

# REFERENCES

—— (1993) *Postmodern Ethics*, Oxford: Blackwell.

—— (1995) *Life in Fragments: Essays in Postmodern Morality*, Oxford: Blackwell.

—— (1998) *Work, Consumerism and the New Poor*, Buckingham: Open University Press.

—— (1999) *In Search of Politics*, Cambridge: Polity Press.

Beck, A. T. (1976) *Cognitive Therapy and the Emotional Disorders*, New York: International University Press.

Beck, A. T., Emery, G. and Greenberg R. (1985) *Anxiety Disorders and Phobias: A Cognitive Perspective*, New York: Basic Books.

Beck, U. (1992) *Risk Society: Towards a New Modernity*, London: Sage Publications.

—— (1994) 'The Reinvention of Politics: Towards a Theory of Reflexive Modernization', in U. Beck, A. Giddens and S. Lash (eds) *Reflexive Modernization: Politics, Tradition and Aesthetics in the Modern Social Order*, Cambridge: Polity Press.

—— (1995) *Ecological Politics in an Age of Risk*, Cambridge: Polity Press.

—— (1997) *The Reinvention of Politics*, Cambridge: Polity Press.

—— (1998) *Democracy Without Enemies*, Cambridge: Polity Press.

—— (1999) *World Risk Society*, Cambridge: Polity Press.

Beck, U. and Beck-Gernsheim, E. (1995) *The Normal Chaos of Love*, Cambridge: Polity Press.

—— (1996) 'Individualization and Precarious Freedoms: Perspectives and Controversies of a Subject-orientated Sociology', in P. Heelas, S. Lash and P. Morris (eds) *Detraditionalization: Critical Reflections on Authority and Identity*, Oxford: Blackwell.

Beck, U., Giddens, A. and Lash, S. (1994) *Reflexive Modernization: Politics, Tradition and Aesthetics in the Modern Social Order*, Cambridge: Polity Press.

Bellaby, P. (1990) 'To Risk or not to Risk? Uses and Limitations of Mary Douglas on Risk Acceptability for Understanding Health and Safety at Work and Road Accidents', *Sociological Review* 38(3): 465–83.

Belle, D. (1991) 'Gender Differences in the Social Moderators of Stress', in A. Monat and R. S. Lazarus (eds) *Stress and Coping: An Anthology*, New York: Columbia University Press.

Berger, P. L., Berger, B. and Kellner, H. (1973) *The Homeless Mind: Modernization and Consciousness*. Harmondsworth: Penguin.

Bernstein, P. L. (1998) *Against the Gods: The Remarkable Story of Risk*, New York: John Wiley & Sons.

Bloch, M. (1961) *Feudal Society*, trans. L. A. Manyon, London: Routledge.

Bocock, R. (1978) *Freud and Modern Society: An Outline and Analysis of Freud's Sociology*, New York: Holmes & Meier Publishers.

Boholm, A. (1996) 'Risk Perception and Social Anthropology: Critique of Cultural Theory', *Ethnos* 61(1–2): 64–84.

Bourdieu, P. (1984) *Distinction: A Social Critique of the Judgement of Taste*, London: Routledge.

Brenot, J., Bonnefous, S. and Marris, C. (1998) 'Testing the Cultural Theory of Risk in France', *Risk Analysis* 18(6): 729–39.

Brewin, C. R. (1996) 'Theoretical Foundations of Cognitive-behaviour Therapy for Anxiety and Depression', *Annual Review of Psychology* 47: 33–57.

# REFERENCES

Briggs, A. (1956) 'From Slaves to Robots', *The New Statesman and Nation*, 23 June, 739.

Brown, G. W., Bifulco, A. and Harris, T. O. (1987) 'Life Events, Vulnerability and Onset of Depression: Some Refinements', *British Journal of Psychology* 150: 30–42.

Brown, G. W. and Harris, T. O. (1978) *Social Origins of Depression: A Study of Psychiatric Disorder in Women*, London: Tavistock Publications.

—— (1989) *Life Events and Illness*, London: Unwin & Hyman.

Brown, G. W., Lemyre, L. and Bifulco, A. (1992) 'Social Factors and Recovery from Anxiety and Depressive Disorders: A Test Specificity', *British Journal of Psychiatry* 161: 55–8.

Brunner, E. and Marmot, M. (1999) 'Social Organization, Stress and Health', in M. Marmot and R. G. Wilkinson (eds) *Social Determinants of Health*, Oxford: Oxford University Press.

Bryant, J., Carveth, R. A. and Brown, D. (1981) 'Television Viewing and Anxiety: An Experimental Examination', *Journal of Communication* 31(1): 106–19.

Byrne, D. (1998) *Complexity Theory and the Social Sciences: An Introduction*, London: Routledge.

Charlton, J., Kelly, S., Dunnell, K., Evans, B. and Jenkins, R. (1993) 'Suicide Deaths in England and Wales: Trends in Factors Associated with Suicide Deaths', *Population Trends* 71(Spring): 34–42.

Clark, L. and Short, J. F. (1993) 'Social Organization and Risk: Some Current Controversies', *Annual Review of Sociology* 19: 375–99.

Cohen, F. (1991) 'Measurement of Coping', in A. Monat and R. S. Lazarus (eds) *Stress and Coping: An Anthology*, New York: Columbia University Press.

Coleman, C. L. (1993) 'The Influence of the Mass Media and Interpersonal Communication on Societal and Personal Risk Judgements', *Communication Research* 20(4): 611–28.

Crook, S. (1991) *Modernist Radicalism and its Aftermath: Foundationalism and Anti-foundationalism in Radical Social Theory*, London: Routledge.

—— (1999) 'Ordering risks', in D. Lupton (ed.) *Risk and Sociocultural Theory: New Directions and Perspectives*, Cambridge: Cambridge University Press.

CSO (Central Statistical Office) (1995) *Social Focus on Women*, London: HMSO.

Culbertson H. M. and Stempel, G. H. (1985) 'Media Malaise: Explaining Personal Optimism and Societal Pessimism about Health Care', *Journal of Communication* 35: 180–90.

Culpitt, I. (1999) *Social Policy and Risk*, London: Sage Publications.

Cutter, S. L. (1993) *Living With Risk: The Geography of Technological Hazards*, London: Edward Arnold.

Cutter, S. L., Tiefenbacher, J. and Solecki, W. D. (1992) 'Engendered Fears: Femininity and Technological Risk Perception', *Industrial Crisis Quarterly* 6: 5–22.

Dahlgren, P. (1988) 'What is the Meaning of This? Viewer's Plural Sense-making of TV News', *Media, Culture and Society* 10: 285–301.

Dake, K. (1991) 'Orienting Dispositions in the Perception of Risk: An Analysis of Contemporary Worldviews and Cultural Biases', *Journal of Cross-Cultural Psychology* 22(1): 61–82.

—— (1992) 'Myths of Nature: Culture and the Social Construction of Risk', *Journal of Social Issues* 48(4): 21–37.

# REFERENCES

Dake, K. and Wildavsky, A. (1990) 'Theories of Risk Perception: Who Fears What and Why?', *Daedalus* 119(4): 41–61.

Dean, M. (1999) 'Risk, Calculable and Incalculable', in D. Lupton (ed.) *Risk and Sociocultural Theory: New Directions and Perspectives*, Cambridge: Cambridge University Press.

Dooley, D., Catalano, R. and Hough, R. (1992) 'Unemployment and Alcohol Disorder in 1910 and 1990: Drift Versus Social Causation', *Journal of Occupational and Organizational Psychology* 64(4): 277–90.

Douglas, M. (1982) 'The Effects of Modernization on Religious Change', *Daedalus* 111(1): 1–19.

—— (1985) *Risk Acceptability According to the Social Sciences*, London: Routledge & Kegan Paul.

—— (1992) *Risk and Blame: Essays in Cultural Theory*, London: Routledge.

—— (1996) *Thought Styles: Critical Essays in Good Taste*, London: Sage Publications.

Douglas, M. and Wildavsky, A. (1982) *Risk and Culture: An Essay in the Selection and Interpretation of Technological and Environmental Dangers*, Berkeley, CA: University of California Press.

Downey, G. and Moen, P. (1987) 'Personal Efficacy, Income and Family Transitions: A Longitudinal Study of Women Heading Households', *Journal of Health and Social Behavior* 21: 260–7.

Drever, F., Whitehead, M. and Roden, M. (1996) 'Current Patterns and Trends in Male Mortality by Social Class (Based on Occupation)', *Population Trends* 86 (Winter): 15–20.

Dunant, S. and Porter, R. (eds) (1996) *The Age of Anxiety*, London: Virago Press.

Dunlap, R. E. and Scarce, R. (1991) 'The Polls – Poll Trends: Environmental Problems and Protection', *Public Opinion Quarterly* 55: 651–72.

Durkheim, E. (1952) *Suicide: A Study in Sociology*, London: Routledge & Kegan Paul.

—— (1964) *The Division of Labour in Society*, New York: The Free Press.

Eckenrode, J. (1991) 'Introduction and Overview', in J. Eckenrode (ed.) *The Social Context of Coping*, New York: Plenum Press.

Edelmann, R. J. (1992) *Anxiety: Theory Research and Intervention in Clinical and Health Psychology*, Chichester: John Wiley & Sons.

Eldridge, J. (1999) 'Risk, Society and the Media: Now you See it, Now you Don't', in G. Philo (ed.) *Message Received*, Harlow: Longman.

Elstad, J. I. (1998) 'The Psycho-social Perspective on Social Inequalities in Health', *Sociology of Health and Illness* 20(5): 598–616.

Ewald, F. (1991) 'Insurance and Risk', in G. Burchell, C. Gordon and P. Miller (eds) *The Foucault Effect: Studies in Governmentality*, London: Harvester Wheatsheaf.

—— (1993) 'Two Infinities of Risk', in B. Massumi (ed.) *The Politics of Everyday Fear*, Minneapolis: University of Minnesota Press.

Eysenck, H. J. (1957) *The Dynamics of Anxiety and Hysteria*, London Routledge.

—— (1967) *The Biological Basis of Personality*, Springfield, IL: Charles C. Thomas.

Farr, R. M. and Moscovici, S. (eds) (1984) *Social Representations*, Cambridge: Cambridge University Press.

Fife-Schaw, C. and Rowe, G. (1996) 'Public Perceptions of Everyday Food Hazards: A Psychometric Study', *Risk Analysis* 16(4): 487–500.

Fischer, W. F. (1970) *Theories of Anxiety*, New York: Harper and Row.

Fischoff, B., Lichtenstein, S., Slovic, P., Derby, S. L. and Keeney, R. L. (1981) *Acceptable Risk*, Cambridge: Cambridge University Press.

Fischoff, B., Slovic, P., Lichtenstein, S., Read, S. and Combs, B. (1978) 'How Safe is Safe Enough? A Psychometric Study of Attitudes Towards Technological Risks and Benefits', *Policy Sciences* 9: 127–52.

Fischoff, B., Watson, S. R. and Hope, C. (1984) 'Defining Risk', *Policy Sciences* 17: 123–39.

Folkman, S., Chesney, M., McKusick, L., Ironson, G., Johnson, D. S. and Goates, J. (1991) 'Translating Coping into an Intervention', in J. Eckendrode (ed.) *The Social Context of Coping*, New York: Plenum Press.

Frank, J. D. (1966) 'Galloping Technology, A New Social Disease', *Journal of Social Issues* 22(4): 1–14.

Franklin, J. (1998) *The Politics of Risk Society*, Cambridge: Polity Press.

Freud, S. (1979) 'Inhibitions, Symptoms and Anxiety', in *On Psychopathology: Inhibitions, Symptoms and Anxiety and Other Works*, trans. J. Strachey, London: Penguin Books.

—— (1985) 'Civilization and its Discontents', in *Civilization, Society and Religion: Group Psychology, Civilization and its Discontents and Other Works*, trans. J. Strachey, London: Penguin Books.

—— (1991) 'Anxiety', in *Introductory Lectures on Psychoanalysis*, trans. J. Strachey, London: Penguin Books.

Freudenberg, W. and Pastor, S. K. (1992) 'Public Responses to Technological Risks: Toward a Sociological Perspective', *Sociological Quarterly* 31(3): 389–412.

Fromm, E. (1942) *The Fear of Freedom*, London: Routledge.

—— (1944) 'Individual and Social Origins of Neurosis', *American Sociological Review* 9(4): 380–4.

—— (1947) *Man for Himself: An Inquiry into the Psychology of Ethics*, New York: Rinehart.

—— (1956) *The Sane Society*, London: Routledge & Kegan Paul.

—— (1970) 'The Crisis of Psychoanalysis', in *The Crisis of Psychoanalysis: Essays on Freud, Marx and Social Psychology*, New York: Henry Holt and Company.

—— (1995) *The Art of Loving*, London: Thorsons.

Fromm, E. and Maccoby, M. (1970) *Social Character in a Mexican Village*, Englewood Cliffs, N J: Prentice-Hall.

Fryer, A. J., Mannuzza, S., Martin, L .Y., Gallops, M. S, Endicott, J., Schleyer, B., Gorman, J. M., Liebowitz, M. R. and Klein, D. F. (1989) 'Reliability of Anxiety Assessment: II.Symptom Agreement', *Archive of General Psychiatry* 46: 1102–10.

Fryer, D. (1995) 'Labour Market Disadvantage, Deprivation and Mental Health: Benefit Agency?', *The Psychologist* June: 265–72.

Fukuyama, F. (1989) 'The End of History?', *The National Interest* 16: 3–18.

Furedi, F. (1997) *Culture of Fear: Risk-Taking and the Morality of Low Expectation*, London: Cassell.

# REFERENCES

Furlong, A. and Cartmel, F. (1997) *Young People and Social Change: Individualization and Risk in Late Modernity*, Buckingham: Open University Press.

Gamson, W. A. and Modigliani, A. (1989) 'Media Discourse and Public Opinion on Nuclear Power: A Constructionist Approach', *American Journal of Sociology* 95(1): 1–37.

Gardner, G. T. and Gould, L. C. (1989) 'Public Perceptions of Risks and Benefits of Technology', *Risk Analysis* 9: 225–42.

Giddens, A. (1989) *Sociology*, Cambridge: Polity Press.

—— (1990) *The Consequences of Modernity*, Cambridge: Polity Press.

—— (1991) *Modernity and Self-Identity: Self and Society in the Late Modern Age*, Cambridge: Polity Press.

—— (1992) *The Transformation of Intimacy*, Cambridge: Polity Press.

—— (1994a) 'Living in a Post-Traditional Society', in U. Beck, A. Giddens and A. Lash (eds) *Reflexive Modernization: Politics, Traditions and Aesthetics in the Modern Social Order*, Cambridge: Polity Press.

—— (1994b) *Beyond Left and Right*, Cambridge: Polity Press.

—— (1998) 'Risk Society: The Context of British Politics', in J. Franklin (ed.) *The Politics of Risk Society*, Cambridge: Polity Press.

Gore, S. and Colten, M. E. (1991) 'Gender, Stress and Distress: Social-Relational Influences', in J. Eckenrode (ed.) *The Social Context of Coping*, New York: Plenum Press.

Gove, W. R. (1972) 'The Relationship between Sex Roles, Mental Illness and Marital Status', *Social Forces* 53: 71–80.

Gove, W. R. and Hee-Choon, S. (1989) 'The Psychological Well-being of Divorced and Widowed Men and Women', *Journal of Family Issues* 10: 122–44.

Gove, W. R., Style, C. B. and Hughes, M. (1990) 'The Effect of Marriage on Well-being of Adults', *Journal of Family Issues* 11: 4–35.

Gove, W. R. and Tudor, J. F. (1973) 'Adult Sex Roles and Mental Illness', *American Journal of Sociology* 78: 812–35.

Graham, H. (1987) 'Women's Smoking and Family Health', *Social Science and Medicine* 25: 47–56.

Graham, J. D. and Wiener, J. B. (eds) (1995) *Risk vs Risk: Tradeoffs in Protecting Health and the Environment*, Cambridge, MA: Harvard University Press.

Gray, J. (1987) *The Psychology of Fear and Stress,* Cambridge: Cambridge University Press.

Gustafson, P. E. (1998) 'Gender Differences in Risk Perception: Theoretical and Methodological Perspectives', *Risk Analysis* 18(6): 805–11.

Habermas, J. (1990) *Moral Consciousness and Communicative Action*, Cambridge: Polity Press.

Hacking, I. (1990) *The Taming of Chance*, Cambridge: Cambridge University Press.

—— (1991) 'How Should we Do the History of Statistics?', in G. Burchell, C. Gordon and P. Miller (eds) *The Foucault Effect: Studies in Governmentality*, London: Harvester Wheatsheaf.

Hall, S. and Jacques, M. (eds) (1989) *New Times: The Changing Face of Politics in the 1990s*, London: Lawrence & Wishart.

# REFERENCES

Hansen, A. (1991) 'The Media and the Social Construction of the Environment', *Media, Culture and Society* 13: 443–58.

Haskey, J. (1995) 'Trends in Marriage and Cohabitation: The Decline in Marriage and the Changing Patterns of Living Partnerships', *Population Trends* 81(Summer): 5–15.

—— (1996) 'The Proportion of Married Couples Who Divorce: Past Patterns and Different Prospects', *Population Trends* 83 (Spring): 25–36.

Hausdorff, D. (1972) *Erich Fromm*, New York: Twayne Publishers.

Heider, F. (1958) *The Psychology of Interpersonal Relations*, New York: John Wiley & Sons.

Henriksen, M. and Heyman, B (1998) 'Being Old and Pregnant', in B. Heyman (ed.) *Risk, Health and Health Care: A Qualitative Approach*, London: Edward Arnold.

Heyman, B. (1998) 'Introduction', in B. Heyman (ed.) *Risk, Health and Health Care: A Qualitative Approach*, London: Edward Arnold.

Heyman, B. and Henriksen, M. (1998) 'Probability and Health Risks', in B. Heyman (ed.) *Risk, Health and Health Care: A Qualitative Approach*, London: Edward Arnold.

Hilgartner, S. and Bosk, C. L. (1988) 'The Rise and Fall of Social Problems: A Public Arenas Model', *American Journal of Sociology* 94(1): 53–78.

Hollway, W. and Jefferson, T. (1997) 'The Risk Society in an Age of Anxiety: Situating Fear of Crime', *British Journal of Sociology* 44(2): 255–66.

Holmes, T. and Rahe, R. (1967) 'The Social Readjustment Rating Scale', *Journal of Psychosomatic Research* 11: 213–18.

Horney, K. (1937) *The Neurotic Personality of Our Time*, London: Routledge & Kegan Paul.

—— (1939) *New Ways in Psychoanalysis*, New York: W. W. Norton.

—— (1946) *Our Inner Conflicts: A Constructive Theory of Neurosis*, London: Routledge & Kegan Paul.

—— (1950) *Neurosis and Human Growth: The Struggle Toward Self-Realization*, New York: W. W. Norton.

Hornig, S. (1990) 'Science Stories: Risk, Power and Perceived Emphasis', *Journalism Quarterly* 67(4): 767–76.

—— (1992) 'Framing Risk: Audience and Reader Factors', *Journalism Quarterly* 69(3): 679–90.

Hughes, M. and Gove, W. R. (1981) 'Living Alone: Social Integration and Mental Health', *American Journal of Sociology* 87: 48–74.

Hutton, W. and Giddens, A. (eds) (2000) *On the Edge: Living with Global Capitalism*, London: Jonathan Cape.

Irwin, A., Simmons, P. and Walker, G. (1999) 'Faulty Environments and Risk Reasoning: The Local Understanding of Industrial Hazards', *Environment and Planning A* 31: 1311–26.

Jackson, R. P. (1989) 'From Profit-sailing to Wage-sailing: Mediterranean Owner-captains and their Crews during the Commercial Revolution', *Journal of Economic History* 18 (Winter): 605–28.

Jarvis, M. J. and Wardle, J. (1999) 'Social Patterning of Individual Health Behaviours: The Case of Cigarette Smoking', in M. Marmot and R. G. Wilkinson (eds) *Social Determinants of Health*, Oxford: Oxford University Press.

# REFERENCES

Jay, M. (1973) *The Dialectical Imagination: A History of the Frankfurt School and the Institute of Social Research 1923–1950*, Berkeley, CA: University of California Press.

—— (1988) *Fin-de Siècle Socialism and Other Essays*, London: Routledge.

Joffe, H. (1999) *Risk and 'The Other'*, Cambridge: Cambridge University Press.

Kaplan, H. B. (1991) 'Social Psychology of the Immune System: A Conceptual Framework and Review of the Literature', *Social Science and Medicine* 33(8): 909–23.

Kasperson, J. X. and Kasperson, R. E. (1996) 'The Social Amplification and Attenuation of Risk', *The Annals of the American Academy of Political and Social Science* 545(May): 95–105.

Kelley, H. H. (1973) 'The Process of Causal Attribution', *American Psychologist* 28: 107–28.

Kelly, S. and Bunting, J. (1998) 'Trends in Suicide in England and Wales, 1982–96', *Population Trends* 92(Summer): 29–41.

Kelly, S., Charlton, J. and Jenkins, R. (1995) 'Suicide Deaths in England and Wales, 1982–92: The Contribution of Occupation and Geography', *Population Trends,* 80 (Summer): 16–25.

Kelly, S., Hertzman, C. and Daniels, M. (1997) 'Searching for the Biological Pathways between Stress and Health', *Annual Review of Public Health* 18: 437–62.

Kessler, R. C. and Cleary, P. D. (1980) 'Social Class and Psychological Distress', *American Sociological Review* 45: 463–78.

Kessler, R. C. and McLeod, J. D. (1984) 'Sex Differences in Vulnerability to Undesirable Life Events', *American Sociological Review* 49: 60–79.

Kierkegaard, S. (1980) *The Concept of Anxiety: A Simple Psychologically Orienting Deliberation on the Dogmatic Issue of Hereditary Sin*, trans. R. Thomte and A. Anderson, Princeton, NJ: Princeton University Press.

Kitzinger, J. (1999) 'A Sociology of Media Power: Key Issues in Audience Reception Research', in G. Philo (ed.) *Message Received*, Harlow: Longman.

Klein, M. (1929) 'Infantile Anxiety Situations Reflected in a Work of Art and in the Creative Impulse', *International Journal of Psycho-Analysis* 10: 436–43.

—— (1946) 'Notes on Some Schizoid Mechanisms', *International Journal of Psycho-Analysis* 27: 99–110.

Kroker, A. and Cook, D. (1988) *The Postmodern Scene: Excremental Culture and Hyper-Aesthetics,* London: Macmillan Education.

Kumar, K. (1993) 'The End of Utopia? The End of Socialism? The End of History?, in K. Kumar and S. Bann (eds) *Utopias and the Millennium*, London: Reaktion Books.

—— (1995) 'Apocalypse, Millennium and Utopia Today', in M. Bull (ed.) *Apocalypse Theory*, Oxford: Basil Blackwell.

Lader, M. (1974) *The Age of Anxiety*, Tunbridge Wells: Institute for Cultural Research.

Ladurie, E. L. R. (1978) *Montaillou: Cathars and Catholics in a French Village 1294–1324*, trans. B. Bray, Harmondsworth: Penguin Books.

Lash, S., Szerszynski, B. and Wynne, B. (eds) (1996) *Risk Environment and Modernity: Towards a New Ecology*, London: Sage Publications.

Lash, S. and Urry, J. (1987) *The End of Organized Capitalism*, Cambridge: Polity Press.

—— (1994) *Economies of Signs and Space*, London: Sage Publications.

Lazarus, R. S. (1999) *Stress and Emotion: A New Synthesis*, London: Free Association Books.

Lazarus, R. S. and Folkman, S. (1984) *Stress, Appraisal and Coping*, New York: Springer.

Leiss, W. (1996) 'Three Phases in the Evolution of Risk Communication Practice', *The Annals of the American Academy of Political and Social Science* 545: 85–94.

Lewis, G. and Pelosi, A. (1990), *Manual of the Revised Clinical Interview Schedule, (CIS-R)*, Calgary, Canada: MRC Institute of Psychiatry.

Locke, E. A. and Taylor, M. S. (1991) 'Stress, Coping and the Meaning of Work', in A. Monat and R. Lazarus (eds) *Stress and Coping: An Anthology*, New York: Columbia University Press.

Luhmann, N. (1993) *Risk: A Sociological Theory*, New York: Aldine de Gruyter.

Lull, J. (1990) *Inside Family Viewing: Ethnographic Research on Television's Audiences*, London: Routledge.

—— (1991) *China Turned On: Television, Reform and Resistance*, London: Routledge.

—— (1999a) *Risk*, London: Routledge.

—— (ed.) (1999b) *Risk and Sociocultural Theory: New Directions and Perspectives*, Cambridge: Cambridge University Press.

MacIntyre, A. (1985) *After Virtue: A Study in Moral Theory,* London: Duckworth.

—— (1988) *Whose Justice? Which Rationality?*, London: Duckworth.

McLeod, J. M., Kosicki, G. M. and Pan, Z. (1991) 'On Understanding and Misunderstanding Media Effects', in J. Curran and M. Gurevitch (eds) *Mass Media and Society*, London: Edward Arnold.

McLuhan, M. (1964) *Understanding Media: The Extensions of Man*, London: Routledge & Kegan Paul.

Maddi, S. R. and Kobasa, S. C. (1991) 'The Development of Hardiness', in A. Monat and R. S. Lazarus (eds) *Stress and Coping: An Anthology*, New York: Columbia University Press.

Mannuzza, S., Fryer, A.J., Martin, L. Y., Gallops, M. S., Endicott, J., Gorman, J., Liebowitz, M. R. and Klein, D. F. (1989) 'Reliability of Anxiety Assessment: I. Diagnostic Agreement' *Archive of General Psychiatry* 46 (December): 1093–101.

Marmot, M. (1999) 'Introduction', in M. Marmot and R. G. Wilkinson (eds) *Social Determinants of Health*, Oxford: Oxford University Press.

Marx, K. (1977) 'Economic and Philosophical Manuscripts', in D. McLellan (ed.) *Karl Marx: Selected Writings*, Oxford: Oxford University Press.

Massumi, B. (1993) 'Everywhere You Want to Be: Introduction to Fear', in B. Massumi (ed.) *The Politics of Everyday Fear,* Minneapolis: University of Minnesota Press.

May, R. (1977) *The Meaning of Anxiety*, New York: W. W. Norton.

Mazur, A. (1981) 'Media Coverage and Public Opinion on Scientific Controversies', *Journal of Communication* 31 (Spring): 106–15.

Meichenbaum, D. (1977) *Cognitive-behavior Modification*, New York: Plenum Press.

Meichenbaum, D. and Cameron, R. (1983) 'Stress Inoculation Training: Toward a General Paradigm for Training Coping Skills', in D. Meichenbaum and M. E. Jeremko (eds) *Stress Reduction and Prevention*, New York: Plenum Press.

# REFERENCES

Mellencamp, P. (1990) 'TV Time Catastrophe, or Beyond the Pleasure Principle of Television', in P. Mellencamp (ed.) *Logics of Television: Essays in Cultural Criticism*, London: BFI Publishing.

Meltzer, H., Gill, B. and Petticrew, M. (1994) 'The Prevalence of Psychiatric Morbidity among Adults Aged 16–64, Living in Private Households, in Great Britain', *OPCS Surveys of Psychiatric Morbidity in Great Britain: Bulletin No.1*, London: OPCS.

Meštrović, S. G. (1991) *The Coming Fin de Siècle: An Application of Durkheim's Sociology to Modernity and Postmodernism*, London: Routledge.

—— (1993) *The Barbarian Temperament*, London: Routledge.

Meyrowitz, J. (1985) *No Sense of Place: The Impact of the Electronic Media on Social Behavior*, New York: Oxford University Press.

Miller, D. and Reilly, J. (1994) *Food Scares in the Media*, Glasgow: Glasgow University Media Unit.

Miller, M. and Rahe, R. (1997) 'Life Changes Scaling for the 1990s', *Journal of Psychosomatic Research* 43(3): 279–92.

Mills, C. W. (1959) *The Sociological Imagination*, New York: Oxford University Press.

Mirowsky, J. and Ross, C. (1986) 'Social Patterns of Distress', *Annual Review of Sociology* 12: 23–45.

—— (1989) *Social Causes of Psychological Distress*, New York: Aldine de Gruyter.

Monat, A. and Lazarus R. S. (eds) (1991) *Stress and Coping: An Anthology*, New York: Columbia University Press.

Morley, D. (1986) *Family Television*, London: Comedia/Routledge.

—— (1992) *Television Audiences and Cultural Studies*, London: Routledge.

Morley, D. and Silverstone, R. (1990) 'Domestic Communication – Technologies and Meanings', *Media, Culture and Society* 12(1): 31–56.

Mowrer, O. H. (1939) 'A Stimulus-response Analysis of Anxiety and its Role as a Reinforcing Agent', *Psychological Review* 46(6): 553–65.

Murdoch, G. (1993) 'Communications and the Constitution of Modernity', *Media, Culture and Society* 15: 521–39.

Nisbet, R. A. (1966) *The Sociological Tradition*, London: Heinemann.

Noble, T. (1982) 'Recent Sociology, Capitalism and the Coming Crisis', *British Journal of Sociology* 33(2): 238–52.

Offe, C. (1996) *Modernity and the State: East, West*, Cambridge: Polity Press.

O'Mahony, P. (ed.) (1999) *Nature, Risk and Responsibility*, London: Macmillan Press.

O'Malley, P. (1996) 'Risk and Responsibility', in A. Barry, T. Osborne and N. Rose (eds) *Foucault and Political Reason: Liberalism, Neo-Liberalism and Rationalities of Government*, London: UCL Press.

ONS (Office for National Statistics) (1998) *Social Trends 28*, London: HMSO.

Pahl, R. (1995) *After Success: Fin-de-Siècle Anxiety and Identity*, Cambridge: Polity Press.

—— (1998) 'Friendship: The Social Glue of Contemporary Society?', in J. Franklin (ed.) *The Politics of Risk Society*, Cambridge: Polity Press.

Pearlin, L. (1989) 'The Sociological Study of Stress', *Journal of Health and Social Behavior* 27: 161–78.

—— (1991) 'The Study of Coping: An Overview of Problems and Directions', in J. Eckenrode (ed.) *The Social Context of Coping*, New York: Plenum Press.

Pilisuk, M. and Acredolo, C. (1988) 'Fear of Technological Hazards: One Concern or Many?', *Social Behavior* 3: 17–24.

Powell, D. and Leiss, W. (1997) *Mad Cows and Mother's Milk: The Perils of Poor Risk Communication*, Montreal and Kingston: McGill-Queen's University Press.

Powell, T. J. and Enright, S. J. (1990) *Anxiety and Stress Management*, London: Routledge.

Rachman, S. (1998) *Anxiety*, Hove: Psychology Press.

Reilly, J. (1999) 'Just Another Food Scare? Public Understanding and the BSE Crisis', in G. Philo (ed.) *Message Received*, Harlow: Longman.

Rickert, J. (1986) 'The Fromm-Marcuse Debate Revisited', *Theory and Society* 15: 351–400.

Riesman, D. (1961) *The Lonely Crowd: A Study of the Changing American Character*, New Haven, CT: Yale University Press.

Riessman, C. K. (1989) 'Life Events, Meaning and Narrative: The Case of Infidelity and Divorce', *Social Science Medicine* 29: 743–51.

—— (1990) *Divorce Talk: Women and Men Make Sense of Personal Relationships*, New Brunswick, NJ: Rutgers University Press.

Robertson, R. (1992) *Globalization: Social Theory and Global Culture*, London: Sage Publications.

de Roover, F. E. (1945) 'Early Examples of Marine Insurance', *Journal of Economic History* 5: 172–200.

Ross, C. and Mirowsky, J. (1979) 'A Comparison of Life-Event-Weighting Schemes: Change, Undesirability, and Effect-Proportional Indices', *Journal of Health and Social Behaviour* 20(June): 166–77.

Ross, L. (1977) 'The Intuitive Psychologist and' his Shortcomings: Distortions in the Attribution Process', in L. Berkowitz (ed.) *Advances in Experimental Social Psychology*, vol. 10, New York: Academic Press.

Royal Society (1983) *Risk Assessment: A Study Group Report*, London: Royal Society.

—— (1992) *Risk: Analysis, Perception and Management*, London: Royal Society.

Schwarz, S. and Thompson, M. (1990) *Divided We Stand: Rethinking Politics, Technology and Social Choice*, Hemel Hempstead: Harvester Wheatsheaf.

Selye, H. (1956) *The Stress of Life*, New York: McGraw-Hill.

—— (1974) *Stress Without Distress*, New York: J.B. Lippincott.

Shaw, C. (1999) '1996-based Population Projections by Legal Marital Status for England and Wales', *Population Trends* 95(Spring): 23–31.

Shaw, C. and Haskey, J. (1999) 'New Estimates and Projections of the Population Cohabiting in England and Wales', *Population Trends* 95(Spring): 7–17.

Silverstone, R. (1994) *Television and Everyday Life,* London: Routledge.

Simmel, G. (1950) 'The Metropolis and Mental Life', in K. H. Wolff (ed.) *The Sociology of Georg Simmel*, New York: The Free Press.

# REFERENCES

—— (1997) 'Culture and Crisis', in D. Frisby and M. Featherstone (eds) *Simmel on Culture*, London: Sage Publications.

Simon, R. W. (1995) 'Gender, Multiple Roles, Role Meaning and Mental Health', *Journal of Health and Social Behavior* 36(2): 182–94.

—— (1997) 'The Meanings Individuals Attach to Role Identities and Their Implications for Mental Health', *Journal of Health and Social Behavior* 38: 256–74.

Simpson, B. (1999) 'Nuclear Fallout: Divorce, Kinship and the Insecurities of Contemporary Life', in J. Vail, J. Wheelock and M. Hill (eds) *Insecure Times: Living with Insecurity in Contemporary Society*, London: Routledge.

Singer, E. and Endreny, P. (1987) 'Reporting Hazards: Their Benefits and Costs', *Journal of Communication* 37(3): 10–26.

Sjoberg, L. (1997) 'Explaining Risk Perception: An Empirical Evaluation of Cultural Theory', *Risk Decision and Policy* 2(2): 113–30.

—— (1998) 'Worry and Risk Perception', *Risk Analysis* 18(1): 85–93.

—— (2000) 'Factors in Risk Perception', *Risk Analysis* 20(1): 1–11.

Skeat, Rev. W. (1910) *An Etymological Dictionary of the English Language*, Oxford: Clarendon.

Skolbekken, J. (1995) 'The Risk Epidemic in Medical Journals', *Social Science and Medicine* 40: 291–305.

Slovic, P. (1987) 'Perception of Risk', *Science* 236(4799): 280–5.

Smail, D. (1984) *Illusion and Reality: The Meaning of Anxiety*, London: J.M. Dent & Sons.

—— (1998) *Taking Care: An Alternative to Therapy*, London: Constable.

—— (1999) *The Origins of Unhappiness: A New Understanding of Personal Distress*, London: Constable.

Spencer, W. J. and Triche, E. (1994) 'Media Constructions of Risk and Safety: Differential Framings of Hazard Events', *Sociological Inquiry* 64(2): 199–213.

Stallings, R. A. (1990) 'Media Discourse and the Social Construction of Risk', *Social Problems* 37(1): 80–95.

Stansfield, S. A. (1999) 'Social Support and Social Cohesion', in M. Marmot and R. G. Wilkinson (eds) *Social Determinants of Health*, Oxford: Oxford University Press.

Steptoe. A. (1991) 'The Links between Stress and Illness', *Journal of Psychosomatic Research* 35(6): 633–44.

Sullivan, H. S. (1953) *The Interpersonal Theory of Psychiatry*, New York: W. W. Norton.

—— (1964) *The Fusion of Psychiatry and Social Science*, New York: W. W. Norton.

Taylor, C. (1989) *Sources of the Self: The Making of the Modern Identity*, Cambridge: Cambridge University Press.

Thoits, P. (1991) 'Gender Differences in Coping with Emotional Distress', in J. Eckenrode (ed.) *The Social Context of Coping*, New York: Plenum Press.

—— (1995a) 'Stress, Coping and Social Support Processes: Where are We? What Next?, *Journal of Health and Social Behavior* Extra Issue: 53–79.

—— (1995b) 'Social Psychology: The Interplay between Sociology and Psychology', *Social Forces*, 73(4): 1231–43.

Thompson, J. B. (1995) *The Media and Modernity: A Social Theory of the Media*, Cambridge: Polity Press.

—— (1996) 'Tradition and Self in a Mediated World', in P. Heelas, S. Lash and P. Morris (eds) *Detraditionalization: Critical Reflections on Authority and Identity*, Oxford: Blackwell Publishers.

Thompson, M., Ellis, R. and Wildavksy, A. (1990) *Cultural Theory*, Boulder, CO: Westview Press.

Tillich, P. (1952) *The Courage To Be*, Glasgow: William Collins.

Turner, R. J. and Avison, W. R. (1992) 'Innovations in the Measurement of Life Stress: Crisis Theory and the Significance of Event Resolution' *Journal of Health and Social Behavior* 33(March): 36–50.

Turner, R. J. and Marino, F. (1994) 'Social Support and Social Structure: A Descriptive Epidemiology', *Journal of Health and Social Behavior* 35: 193–212.

Turner R. J. and Roszell, P. (1994) 'Psychosocial Resources and the Stress Process', in W. R. Avison and I. H. Gotlib (eds) *Stress and Mental Health: Contemporary Issues and Prospects for the Future*, New York: Plenum Press.

Turner R. J, Wheaton, B. and Donald, L. (1995) 'The Epidemiology of Social Stress', *The American Sociological Review* 60(February): 104–25.

Tyler, T. T. and Cook, F. L. (1984) 'The Mass Media and Judgements of Risk: Distinguishing Impact on Personal and Societal Level Judgements', *Journal of Personality and Social Psychology* 47(4): 693–708.

Ulbrich, P. M., Warheit, G. J. and Zimmerman, R. S. (1989) 'Race, Socioeconomic Status, and Psychological Distress: An Examination of Differential Vulnerability', *Journal of Health and Social Behavior* 30: 131–46.

Vail, J., Wheelock, J. and Hill, M. (eds) (1999) *Insecure Times: Living with Insecurity in Contemporary Society*, London: Routledge.

Vaillant, G. E. (1977) *Adaption to Life*, Boston: Little, Brown.

Wadsworth, M. (1999) 'Early Life', in M. Marmot and R. G. Wilkinson (eds) *Social Determinants of Health*, Oxford: Oxford University Press.

Weber, M. (1948) 'Science as a Vocation', in H. H. Gerth and C. W. Mills (eds) *From Max Weber: Essays in Sociology,* London: Routledge.

—— (1949) *The Methodology of the Social Sciences*, New York: The Free Press.

—— (1958) *The Protestant Ethic and the Spirit of Capitalism*, New York: Charles Scribner's Sons.

Weinstein, N. D. (1980) 'Unrealistic Optimism about Future Life Events', *Journal of Personality and Social Psychology* 39(2): 186–218.

—— (1982) 'Unrealistic Optimism about Susceptibility to Health Problems', *Journal of Behavioral Medicine* 5: 441–60.

—— (1987) 'Unrealistic Optimism about Susceptibility to Health Problems: Conclusions from a Community Wide Sample', *Journal of Behavioral Medicine* 10: 481–95.

Wheelock, J. (1999) 'Fear or Opportunity? Insecurity in Employment', in J. Vail, J. Wheelock and M. Hill (eds) *Insecure Times: Living with Insecurity in Contemporary Society*, London: Routledge.

# REFERENCES

WHO (World Health Organization) (1993a) *Composite International Diagnostic Interview –
Version 1.1*, Geneva: WHO.

—— (1993b) *The ICD-10 Classification of Mental and Behavioural Disorders: Diagnostic
Criteria for Research*, Geneva: WHO.

Wilkins, L. and Patterson, P. (1987) 'Risk Analysis and the Construction of News', *Journal of
Communication* 37(3): 80–92.

Wilkinson, I. (1999) 'Where is the Novelty in our Current Age of Anxiety?', *European Journal
of Social Theory* 2(4): 445–67.

—— (2001) 'Social Perceptions of Risk Perception: At Once Indispensable and Insufficient',
*Current Sociology* 49(1): 1–21.

Wilkinson, R. G. (1996) *Unhealthy Societies: The Afflictions of Inequality*, London: Routledge.

—— (1999) 'Putting the Picture Together: Prosperity, Redistribution, Health, and Welfare' in
M. Marmot and R. G. Wilkinson (eds) *Social Determinants of Health*, Oxford: Oxford
University Press.

Wilkinson, R. G., Kawachi, I. and Kennedy, B. (1998) 'Mortality, the Social Environment,
Crime and Violence', *Sociology of Health and Illness* 20(5): 578–97.

Williams, R. (1958) *Culture and Society 1780–1950*, Harmondsworth: Penguin Books.

—— (1961) *The Long Revolution*, Harmondsworth: Penguin Books.

Wober, M. and Gunter, B. (1982) 'Television and Personal Threat: Fact or Artefact? A British
Survey', *British Journal of Social Psychology* 21: 239–47.

Young, K. (1990) 'Living Under Threat', in R. Jowell, S. Witherspoon and L. Brook (eds)
*British Social Attitudes – 7th Report*, Aldershot: Gower.

# Index

# INDEX

# INDEX

# INDEX

# INDEX